KIDNEY DISEASE AND
LABORATORY MEDICINE

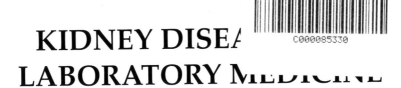

Edmund Lamb BSc, MSc, PhD, FRCPath
Consultant Clinical Scientist, East Kent Hospitals University NHS
Foundation Trust

Michael Delaney BSc, MD, FRCP
Consultant Nephrologist, East Kent Hospitals University NHS
Foundation Trust

Editors:
Marta Lapsley MD, FRCPath
Consultant Chemical Pathologist, Epsom General Hospital

Beverley Harris BSc, MSc, FRCPath
Principal Clinical Scientist, Royal United Hospital, Bath

ACB VENTURE PUBLICATIONS
with generous support from
SIEMENS HEALTHCARE DIAGNOSTICS LTD. AND SCIPAC

ACB VENTURE PUBLICATIONS
Chairman - Ruth Lapworth

British Library Cataloguing in Publication Data

A catalogue record for the book is available from the British Library

ISBN 978-0-902429-45-1, EAN 9780902429451, ACB Venture Publications

Printed by Piggotts Black Bear (Cambridge) Limited

Cover and illustrations by Alan Sherwood, Aspire Design Studios,
London

© Copyright 2009. Association for Clinical Biochemistry, 130-132 Tooley St, London
SE1 2TU

All rights reserved. No part of this publication may be reproduced, stored in a retrieval
system or transmitted in any form or by any means electronic, mechanical, photo-
copying, recording or otherwise, without written permission from the publisher.

Preface

The kidneys have complex and diverse functions, having a critical role in salt, water and acid-base homeostasis and in excretion of waste products of metabolism. In addition, the kidney's endocrine role in the production of activated vitamin D and erythropoietin, means that disease processes that compromise function can result in a variety of pathological manifestations. In contrast to many other disorders, the onset of kidney disease is often insidious and early detection relies heavily on laboratory testing. Conversely, episodes of acute kidney injury may precipitate life threatening emergencies very rapidly and succesful management relies on meticulous attention to laboratory reports with appropriate interpretation of the data.

Renal medicine and chemical diagnostics have long been intertwined: well known descriptions of albuminuria date back to Richard Bright's report of albuminous nephritis (Bright's disease) in the early nineteenth century, although much earlier descriptions have also been proposed as probable nephritis. The increasing use of renal dialysis and transplantation during the latter half of the twentieth century was heavily underpinned by laboratory support. Recently, the importance of chronic kidney disease as a public health issue and the requirement for early identification of kidney disease has been more widely appreciated with the development of a series of expert opinion-based clinical guidelines. Laboratory testing is at the forefront of these initiatives.

Understanding the role of the laboratory in supporting renal medicine is essential to the function of clinical scientists. We hope that the collaboration between clinical nephrologist and scientist in this book will provide the reader with a clear understanding of the physiology and diverse pathophysiology of the kidney, as well as the basic principles underlying the modern approrach to the management of kidney diseases. Throughout, we have placed an emphasis on how and when laboratory testing should be used to underpin this branch of medicine.

We would like to thank ACB Venture Publications for inviting us to write this book and in particular Dr Marta Lapsley and Miss Beverley Harris for editorial support and Dr Roy Sherwood for design and layout. Preparing this book has been an enjoyable experience and we hope that readers will find it useful.

Edmund Lamb
Michael Delaney
December 2008

Acknowledgements

The authors are grateful to the following for permission to reproduce or adapt material for certain figures used in this publication:

American Journal of Kidney Disease. Foley RN, Parfrey PS, Sarnak MJ. Am J Kidney Dis 1998; **32 (suppl 3):** S112-S119 (Figure 6.1).

American Society for Nephrology, Soriano JR. J Am Soc Nephrol 2002; **13:** 2160-70 (Figures 1.7 and 1.9), Froissart M, *et al*. J Am Soc Nephrol 2005; **16:** 763-73 (Figure 3.9), Bonventre J and Weinberg JM. J Am Soc Nephrol 2003; **14:** 2199-2210 (Figure 4.2) and Chunsun D *et al*. J Am Soc Nephrol 2006; **17:** 2164-75 (Figure 5.5).

Annals of Internal Medicine. Levey AS, *et al*. Ann Intern Med 1999; **130:** 461-70 (Figure 3.7).

Association for Clinical Biochemistry. Sayer JA and Pearce SHS. Ann Clin Biochem 2001; **38:** 459-470 (Figures 1.5 and 1.6).

Nancy Lou Riccio. Brenner BM and Beeuwkes R, III: Hospital Practice **13:** 35-46, July 1978 (Figure 1.3).

Saunders. Brenner and Rector's The Kidney, 7th edition, 2004, Chapter 1, pp 3-72. (Figure 1 .1) and Chapter 5, pp 231-260 (Figure 1.4).

UKNEQAS. Edinburgh, distribution 95, September 2006 (Figure 6.5).

UK Transplant. (Figure 7.8).

United Kingdom Renal Registry. (Figures 8.3 & 8.4).

United States Renal Data System. Excerpts from the USRDS 2006 Annual Data Report. Am J Kidney Dis 2007; **49:** S1-S296 (suppl 1) (Figure 2.1).

Contents

Important notice

Although ACB Venture Publications has made every effort to ensure the accuracy of the information contained in this book, the responsibility for the patient is ultimately that of the medical practitioner ordering or performing/supervising the investigations. All drugs and intravenous fluids must be prescribed by a registered medical practitioner and administered by an individual authorised to do so. The publishers, authors and editors do not assume any liability for any injury and/or damage to persons or property arising from this publication.

Chapter 1

Renal anatomy and physiology

The basic anatomy and physiology of the kidneys are described in this chapter as a foundation to understanding the pathophysiology of disease and the rationale for diagnostic and management strategies in kidney disease.

Anatomy

Gross anatomy

The kidneys are located in the retroperitoneal space, extending from the level of the lower part of the 11th thoracic vertebra to the upper portion of the 3rd lumbar vertebra; the right kidney is situated slightly lower than the left. Adult kidneys are about 12 cm long and weigh about 150 g in men and 135 g in women.

Blood supply

In the majority of cases each kidney receives its blood supply from a single renal artery derived from the abdominal aorta, although multiple renal arteries are common. The renal artery divides into posterior and anterior elements and ultimately into the afferent arterioles, which expand into the highly specialised capillary bed that forms the glomerulus. Figure 1.1 shows a glomerulus with its afferent arteriole taking its origin from an interlobular artery at lower left. The capillaries of the glomerulus rejoin to form the efferent arteriole, which then forms the capillary plexuses as well as the elongated vessels (the vasa recta) that pass around the remaining parts of the nephron, the proximal and distal tubules, the loop of Henle, and collecting duct. The efferent arteriole then merges with renal venules to form the renal veins, which emerge into the inferior vena cava. In the adult, the kidneys receive approximately 25% of the cardiac output, about 90% of which supplies the renal cortex, maintaining the highly active tubular cells.

Nephron

The functional unit of the kidney is the nephron. Each kidney contains between 0.4 and 1.2 million nephrons. The number of nephrons that an individual is born with (the 'nephron dose') may determine that individual's susceptibility to renal injury. Two main nephron populations exist (short and long nephrons) depending on the position of the glomerulus within the cortex (Figure 1.2). The nephron consists of a glomerulus, proximal tubule, loop of Henle, distal tubule, and collecting duct. The collecting ducts ultimately combine to develop into the renal calyces, where the urine collects before passing along the ureter and into the bladder. The kidney is divided into several lobes. The outer region of each lobe, the cortex, consists of most of the glomeruli and the proximal and distal tubules. The cortex surrounds an inner region, the medulla, which is further divided into a number of conical areas known as the renal pyramids, the apices of which extend toward the renal pelvis, forming papillae. There are visible striations in the renal pyramids (the 'medullary rays') which contain the straight tubular elements (i.e. collecting ducts and the loops of Henle with associated blood vessels (the vasa recta)). The central hilus is where blood vessels, lymphatics, and the renal pelvis (containing the ureter) join the kidney.

Scanning electron micrograph of a cast of a glomerulus

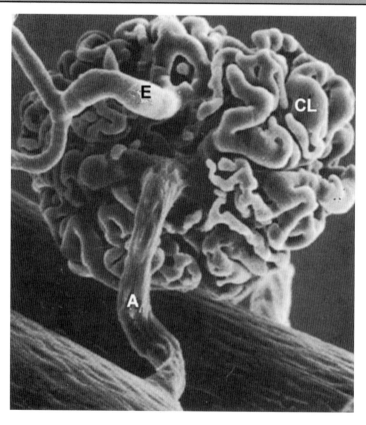

Figure 1.1 Scanning electron micrograph of a cast of a glomerulus (magnification x300). A, afferent arteriole; CL, capillary loops; E, efferent arteriole. (Courtesy of Waykin Nopanitaya, PhD). Reproduced with permission from Madsen KM, Tisher CC. Anatomy of the Kidney. In: Brenner BM. Brenner and Rector's The Kidney, 7th edition, Saunders, Philadelphia, 2004, Chapter 1, pp 3-72.

The nephron

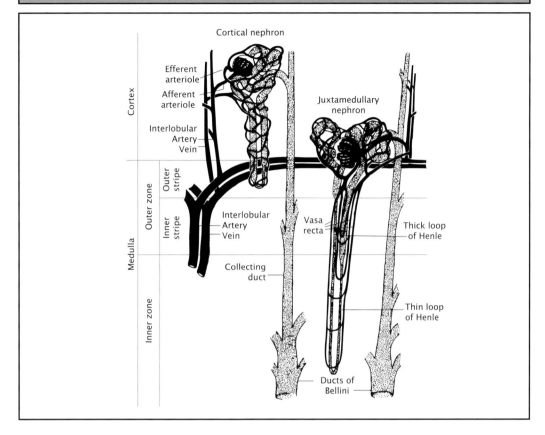

Figure 1.2 Diagrammatic representation of the nephron, the functional unit of the kidney, illustrating the anatomical and vascular arrangements.

GLOMERULUS (PLATES 1-3)

The glomerulus (renal corpuscle) is formed from a specialised capillary network (Figure 1.1) enclosed within a Bowman's capsule. Each capillary develops into approximately 40 glomerular loops some 200 µm in size consisting of a variety of different cell types (endothelial, epithelial and mesangial) supported on the glomerular basement membrane (Figure 1.3); together these form the glomerular filtration barrier. The capillary endothelial cells are in contact with each other, but between these cells there are many circular fenestrations (pores) with diameters of between 70 and 100 nm. The fenestrations are lined with a surface coating of negatively charged glycoproteins about 12 nm thick, which allows virtually free access of plasma to the basement membrane. The latter forms the only continuous barrier between the capillary blood and glomerular filtrate.

The glomerular cells and the glomerular filtration barrier

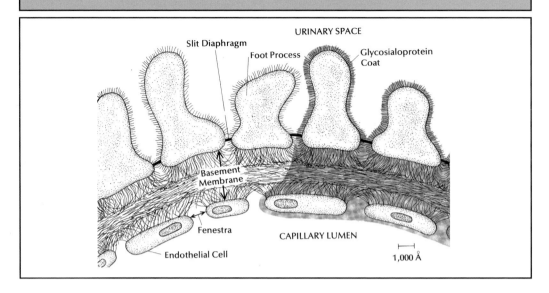

Figure 1.3 The glomerular cells and the glomerular filtration barrier. The shaded area represents the distribution of negatively charged glycosialoproteins. Reproduced from Brenner BM, Beeuwkes R, III: The kidney in health and disease: III. The renal circulations. Hospital Practice **13**: 35-46, July 1978 with permission of the artist (Nancy Lou Riccio).

The visceral epithelial cells lining the urinary side of the glomerular basement membrane (Figure 1.3) are called podocytes and have an unusual octopus-like structure in that they have a large number of extensions or foot processes that are embedded in the basement membrane. The foot processes from adjacent podocytes are interdigitated to form filtration slits, which are covered by a loose, highly hydrated anionic mucopolysaccharide gel that is rich in sialic acid. The resulting structure is relatively impermeable to molecules larger than 60 kDa. The podocytes are thought to be responsible, in part, for the synthesis and mainte-nance of the basement membrane. Bowman's capsule is lined by parietal epithe-lial cells. Between the visceral and parietal epithelial cells is a narrow cavity called Bowman's space (urinary space).

The basement membrane (Figure 1.3) is approximately 300 nm thick in adult humans and consists of three distinct layers: the lamina rara interna, the darker lamina densa and the lamina rara externa. The lamina densa consists of a close feltwork of fine, mainly type IV, collagen fibrils (each 3-5 nm thick) embedded in a gel-like matrix of glycoproteins and proteoglycans. This forms the main size discriminant barrier to protein passage into the tubular lumen. The other two layers of the basement membrane are rich in negatively charged polyanionic glycoproteins such as heparan sulphate; these form the main charge discriminant barrier to the passage of circulating polyanions (e.g. albumin).

The mesangial cells are found in the central part of the glomerulus between and within the capillary loops suspended in a matrix that they synthesise. They are phagocytic and participate in the clearance of macromolecules (e.g. circulating antigen-antibody complexes). Mesangial cells are rich in myofilaments and provide structural support to the glomerular capillary loops. Additionally, they can contract in response to a variety of stimuli (e.g. angiotensin II (AII) and vaso-pressin) and have a significant effect on the glomerular filtration rate (GFR) by reducing the available filtration surface.

PROXIMAL TUBULE

Bowman's capsule forms the beginning of the tightly coiled, proximal convoluted tubule (pars convoluta) that, on its progress toward the renal medulla, becomes straightened and is then called the pars recta. The human proximal tubule is about 14 mm long. The epithelial cells lining the convoluted section are cuboidal/columnar cells with a luminal brush border consisting of millions of microvilli that enormously expand the surface area for absorption of tubular fluid. Ultrastructurally there are three main segments, S1, S2, and S3, which consist of very different cell types characterised by different types of brush border, density of mitochondria, and degree of cellular interdigitation. There are also functional differences, as demonstrated by the region-specific nephrotoxicity of certain drugs or metals (e.g. mercury is an S3-segment-specific toxin). Fluid reab-sorption in the S3 segment is significantly less than in the S1 and S2 segments. The transition from S1 to S2 is gradual and occurs in the latter part of the pars convo-luta. The S2 to S3 transition occurs in the initial portion of the pars recta.

LOOP OF HENLE

The pars recta drains into the descending thin limb of the loop of Henle, which, after passing through a hairpin loop, becomes first the thin ascending limb and then the thick ascending limb. The cells of the thin ascending limb are very similar to those in the descending thin limb (with little brush border, flattened and inter-digitated), but there are important differences in their permeability to water and in their capability for active transport. The thick ascending limb is lined with cuboidal/columnar cells similar in size to those in the proximal tubule, but they do not possess a brush border. At the end of the thick ascending limb, near where it re-enters the cortex, and closely associated with the glomerulus and the efferent arteriole, there is a cluster of cells known as the macula densa (see p6). The main role of the loop of Henle is to provide the ability to generate a concentrated urine, hypertonic with respect to plasma.

DISTAL TUBULE

The distal tubule includes the thick ascending limb of the loop of Henle, the macula densa and the distal convoluted tubule (pars convoluta). These form three morphologically and functionally distinct segments.

COLLECTING DUCT

The collecting ducts are functionally part of the nephron but are embryologically distinct from it and are formed from approximately six distal tubules. These are successively joined by other tubules to form a duct of Bellini, which ultimately drains into a renal calyx. The cells lining the collecting duct (principal cells) are cuboidal and have a less granular cytoplasm than those of the proximal tubule, although there are a number of interspersed cells (intercalated cells) with a more granular cytoplasm.

Other regions of the kidney

JUXTAGLOMERULAR APPARATUS

Where the thick ascending limb of the loop of Henle passes very close to the glomerulus of its own nephron, the cells of the tubule and the afferent arteriole show regional specialisation. The tubule forms the macula densa and the arteriolar cells are filled with granules (containing renin) and are innervated with sympathetic nerve fibres. This area is called the juxtaglomerular apparatus (JGA). The JGA plays an important part in maintaining systemic blood pressure through regulation of the circulating intravascular blood volume and sodium concentration. The proteolytic enzyme renin is released primarily in response to decreased afferent arteriolar pressure and decreased intraluminal sodium delivery to the macula densa. Renin release from the macula densa is also influenced by renal cortical prostaglandins (predominantly PGI_2) and the sympathetic nervous system. The released renin then acts on the plasma protein angiotensinogen to generate angiotensin I. This is converted in the lungs by angiotensin converting enzyme (ACE) to the potent vasoconstrictor and stimulator of aldosterone release, AII. The vasoconstriction and aldosterone release (with increased distal tubular sodium retention) act in concert with the other action of AII, to increase the release of antidiuretic hormone (ADH, vasopressin), thereby increasing proximal tubular sodium reabsorption, intravascular volume, and pressure. AII also has an inhibitory effect on renin release as part of a negative feedback loop.

RENAL INTERSTITIUM

The interstitium consists of a variety of cell types in an extracellular matrix of glycosaminoglycans. It constitutes 7-9% by volume of the cortex and a larger proportion of the medulla. The interstitium provides structural support, helps stabilise the high osmotic gradient essential to the countercurrent mechanism involved in the generation of a hyperosmotic urine and is also a site of hormone production (e.g. erythropoietin (EPO) and prostaglandins).

Kidney function

The kidneys have a range of functions, but their primary role is to maintain the optimal chemical composition of the blood and the interstitial and intracellular fluids throughout the body, i.e. to maintain homeostasis. The mechanisms of differential reabsorption and secretion, located in the tubule of a nephron, are the effectors of regulation. The mechanisms operate under a complex system of control in which both extrarenal and intrarenal humoral factors participate.

Excretory and reabsorptive functions

The excretory function of the kidney rids the body of many of the undesirable end products of metabolism (e.g. the non-protein nitrogenous compounds urea, creatinine and uric acid) as well as any excess of inorganic substances ingested in the diet (e.g. sodium, potassium, chloride, calcium, phosphate, magnesium and sulphate). Daily intake of water may also exceed the requirements of the body and under such circumstances becomes additional waste material requiring excretion. In order to achieve excretion of the metabolic wastes and the ingested surpluses without disrupting homeostasis, the kidneys must exercise their excretory and reabsorptive functions in the production of urine.

Formation of urine

The first step in urine formation is filtration of plasma at the glomeruli. A net filtration pressure of about 17 mmHg in the capillary bed drives the filtrate through the glomerular membrane. Filtered fluid is believed to traverse the capillary wall via an extracellular route; that is through endothelial fenestrae, basement membrane, and slit diaphragms (Figure 1.3). The filtrate is called an ultrafiltrate because its composition is essentially the same as that of plasma, but with a notable reduction in molecules of molecular weight exceeding 15 kDa. Each nephron produces about 100 μL of ultrafiltrate per day. Overall, approximately 200 L of ultrafiltrate pass through the glomeruli in 24 h. Tubular reabsorption of solutes and water from the ultrafiltrate reduces the total urine volume excreted and modifies its composition.

Different regions of the tubule specialise in certain functions. The proximal tubule is the most metabolically active part of the nephron, facilitating the reabsorption of 60 to 80% of the glomerular filtrate volume, including 70% of the filtered load of sodium and chloride, most of the potassium, bicarbonate, phosphate and sulphate, as well as secreting 90% of the hydrogen ion excreted by the kidney. Glucose is virtually completely reabsorbed in the proximal tubule by a passive, but sodium-dependent, process which is saturated at a blood glucose concentration of about 10 mmol/L. Uric acid is reabsorbed in the proximal tubule by a passive sodium-dependent mechanism, but there is also an active secretory mechanism. Creatinine is also secreted at a rate of approximately 2.5 μmol/min.

In the loops of Henle, chloride and more sodium without water are reabsorbed, generating dilute urine. Water reabsorption in the more distal tubules and collecting ducts is then regulated by ADH. In the distal tubule, secretion is the prominent activity; organic ions, potassium ions, and hydrogen ions are transported from the blood in the efferent arteriole into the tubular fluid.

The final product, urine, is defined as a fluid excreted by the kidneys, passed through the ureters, stored in the bladder, and discharged through the urethra. In health, it is sterile and clear, and has an amber colour, a slightly acid pH (approximately pH 5.0 to 6.0) and a characteristic odour. In addition to dissolved compounds it contains a number of cellular fragments, complete cells, proteinaceous casts, and crystals (formed elements). Urination, also termed micturition, is the discharge of urine. In normal adults, adequate homeostasis can be maintained with a urine output of about 500 mL/24 h. Alterations in urinary output are described as anuria (< 100 mL/24 h), oliguria (< 400 mL/24 h), or polyuria (> 3 L/24 h or > 50 mL/kg body weight/24 h).

Electrolyte homeostasis
Transport of solutes and water occurs both across and between the tubular epithelial cells. Paracellular (between cell) movement is driven predominantly by concentration, osmotic, or electrical gradients. Transport can be both active (energy requiring) or passive, but many of the so-called passive transport processes are secondary (or tertiary) to active transport processes. The most important of these in the nephron is sodium-potassium adenosine triphosphatase (Na^+-K^+-ATPase), which is located on the basolateral membranes of the tubulo-epithelial cells. This enzymatic transporter accounts for much of renal oxygen consumption and drives over 99% of renal sodium reabsorption. The distinction between primary, secondary and tertiary active transport processes is illustrated in Figure 1.4 using Na^+-K^+-ATPase as the example. Primary active transporters use the energy derived from hydrolysis of ATP to power the transport of solutes across the plasma membrane against their electrochemical gradients. Secondary active transporters utilise the energy in the electrochemical gradient (in this example, Na^+) generated by the primary active transport process to drive the influx or efflux of a coupled solute. Tertiary active transport links the transport of a solute (in this example, Cl^-) to the gradient (in this case, H^+) created by the secondary active transport process. Other examples of primary active transport mechanisms are Ca^{2+}-ATPase, H^+-ATPase and H^+-K^+-ATPase. These enzymes

establish ionic gradients, polarising cell membranes and thus driving secondary transport processes. All known transport processes involve receptor or mediator molecules, the activity of many of which is regulated by phosphorylation facilitated by protein kinase C or A. Their renal distribution has been shown to correlate with the known regional functional activities, but the same transporters, or isoforms of them, can be found in other tissues, particularly the digestive tract.

Active transport processes in renal epithelial cells

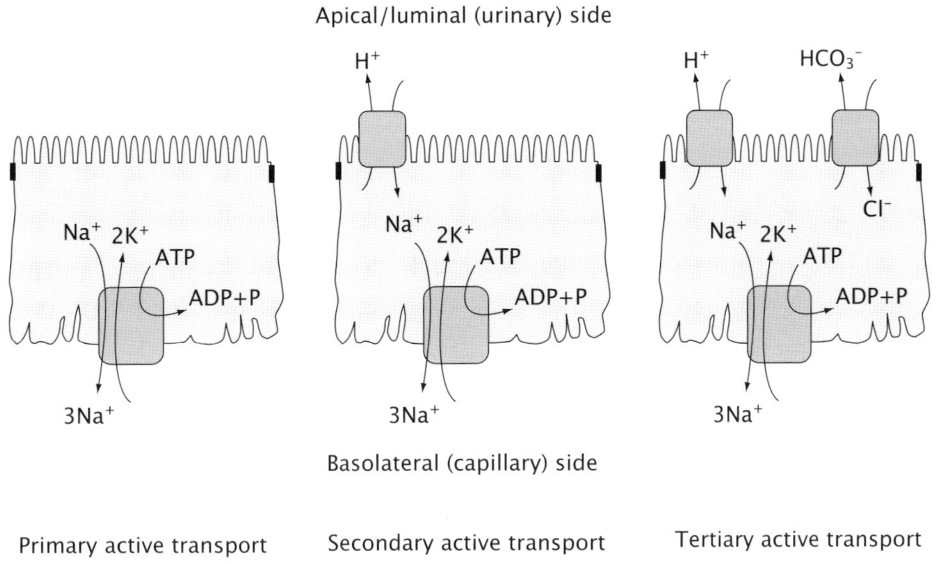

Figure 1.4 Active transport processes in renal epithelial cells. Models of three epithelial cells are shown to illustrate the various modes of active transport. The apical membrane is shown at the top and the basolateral membrane at the bottom. Reproduced with permission from Kone BC. The Metabolic Basis of Solute Transport. In: Brenner BM. Brenner and Rector's The Kidney, 7th edition, Saunders, Philadelphia, 2004, Chapter 5, pp 231-260.

Renal epithelial cell membranes also contain proteins that act as ion channels. For example, there is one for sodium that is closed by amiloride and modulated by hormones such as atrial natriuretic peptide (ANP). Ion channels enable much faster rates of transport than ATPases but are relatively fewer in number, there being approximately 100 sodium and chloride channels compared with 10^7 Na^+-K^+-ATPase molecules per cell. There is a complex interplay between the tubular transport systems regulating individual electrolytes. For simplicity, we have considered electrolytes individually and have restricted our discussion to the systems of major physiological, pharmacological and pathological significance.

SODIUM

Sodium reabsorption is required for the reabsorption of water and many solutes. The proximal tubule is highly permeable to sodium, and the net flux of reabsorption from the tubular lumen is achieved against a high backflux, particularly from paracellular movement. Approximately 60% of filtered sodium is reabsorbed in the proximal tubule in an energy-dependent manner, driven by basolateral Na^+-K^+-ATPase pumps. Most of the sodium entering proximal tubular cells does so in exchange for hydrogen ion secretion, facilitated by apical sodium-hydrogen exchangers. This, in turn, permits bicarbonate reabsorption (see below). A variety of apical sodium cotransporters also allow for reabsorption of other organic and inorganic solutes (e.g. chloride, calcium, phosphate, bicarbonate, sulphate, glucose, urea, and amino acids). Sodium transport activity is regulated by many factors, including protein kinase-dependent phosphorylation, which can increase both activity and channel numbers.

A further 30% of filtered sodium is reabsorbed in the thick ascending limb of the loop of Henle. This is achieved by an apical, bumetanide-sensitive, 130 kDa, electroneutral, Na^+-K^+-$2Cl^-$ cotransporter (NKCC2), itself driven by a favourable inward gradient (i.e. low intracellular sodium and chloride concentrations) generated by the basolateral Na^+-K^+-ATPase pump and the basolateral chloride channel CLC-Kb (Figure 1.5). The availability of potassium is rate limiting for NKCC2, so potassium entering the cell is recycled back to the lumen via the ROMK1 potassium channel. This potassium movement is electrogenic and drives paracellular reabsorption of magnesium and calcium via paracellin-1. NKCC2 is a kidney-specific member of a class of such channels found throughout secretory epithelia. Activation of these cotransporters appears, in part, to be as a result of cell shrinkage. The distal convoluted tubule reabsorbs 5-8% of sodium via the thiazide-sensitive Na^+-Cl^- cotransporter (NCCT). Final sodium balance is achieved in the collecting duct via principal cell selective amiloride-sensitive, apical sodium channels (ENaCs) in exchange for potassium (Figure 1.6). ENaCs are controlled, in part, by the effects of aldosterone on the mineralocorticoid receptor (MR), with hyperaldosteronism producing an increase in channel activity. Cortisol, if permitted, will also bind to the MR, but a degree of specificity is maintained by 11β-hydroxysteroid dehydrogenase (11β-HSD), which inactivates cortisol to cortisone. Sodium uptake drives potassium secretion from principal cells and proton secretion from α-intercalated cells. Liquorice causes hypertension and a hypokalaemic metabolic alkalosis by inactivating 11β-HSD, allowing cortisol to act as a mineralocorticoid. Mutations of ENaC (Liddle's syndrome, pseudohypoaldosteronism type Ia) or the MR (pseudohypoaldosteronism type Ib) cause inherited tubulopathies (see Chapter 5).

Solute reabsorption in the thick ascending limb of the loop of Henle

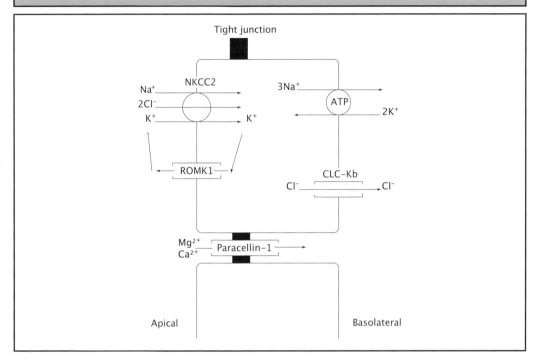

Figure 1.5 Major pathways of solute reabsorption in the thick ascending limb of the loop of Henle. Mutations in either NKCC2, ROMK1 or CLC-Kb (or its associated protein barttin) cause Bartter's syndrome. Mutations in paracellin-1 lead to disruption of this paracellular pathway and the tubular disease known as hypomagnesaemic hypercalciuric nephrolithiasis (see Chapter 5). Reproduced with permission from Sayer JA, Pearce SHS. Diagnosis and clinical biochemistry of inherited tubulopathies. Ann Clin Biochem 2001; **38**: 459-470.

POTASSIUM

Approximately 90% of daily potassium loss occurs via renal elimination. Potassium is freely filtered across the glomerulus and normally almost completely reabsorbed in the proximal tubule. However, most regulatory mechanisms affect the loop of Henle, the distal tubule and the collecting duct. Indeed, urinary losses can exceed filtered load, indicating the importance of distal secretion. Determinants of urinary potassium loss are dietary intake of potassium, acid-base disturbances (acidosis reduces potassium secretion and *vice versa*), plasma potassium concentration, circulating ADH concentration, tubular flow rate and aldosterone secretion (enhances potassium loss and increases sodium retention). Potassium ions are actively accumulated within tubular cells as a result of basolateral Na^+-K^+-ATPase activity, resulting in elevation of intracellular potassium concentration above its electrochemical equilibrium. Several types of potassium channels exist which have a range of functions: (1) maintenance of a negative resting cell membrane potential, (2) regulation of intracellular volume, (3) recycling of potassium across apical and basolateral membranes to supply NKCC2 and enable sodium reabsorption, and (4) potassium secretion in the cortical collecting tubule. As mentioned above, potassium is reabsorbed with sodium by the NKCC2 in the thick ascending limb of the loop of Henle, but is recycled back into the lumen by the potassium-secreting channel ROMK1 (Figure 1.5). ROMK1 is a pH-sensitive, membrane spanning protein with several serine residues; at least two of these residues require phosphorylation by protein kinase A for the channel to be active. In the principal cells of the collecting duct, sodium reabsorption via ENaC is accompanied by movement of potassium into the lumen through potassium channels or a potassium chloride symporter (Figure 1.6).

Solute reabsorption in the collecting duct

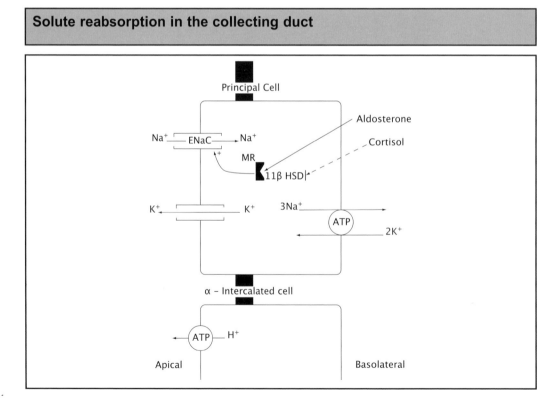

Figure 1.6 Major pathways of solute reabsorption in the collecting duct. Reproduced with permission from Sayer JA, Pearce SHS. Diagnosis and clinical biochemistry of inherited tubulopathies. Ann Clin Biochem 2001; **38**: 459-470.

CHLORIDE

In the early (S1) proximal tubule, avid reabsorption of glucose and amino acids (in conjunction with sodium) generates a negative intra-luminal potential. This drives movement of chloride out of the lumen via a paracellular route. Preferential S1 reabsorption of glucose, amino acids and bicarbonate results in an increase in the luminal chloride concentration; as fluid enters the S2 and S3 segments of the proximal tubule, this enables reabsorption of chloride (in association with sodium) by passive diffusion. Proximal chloride reabsorption is also achieved by active electroneutral sodium chloride uptake and by a secondary active process involving a Na^+/H^+ exchanger. Other chloride exchangers (e.g. chloride/formate exchanger) are probably also important. In the thick ascending limb of the loop of Henle, chloride is reabsorbed in association with sodium via NKCC2; the concentration gradient is maintained by passive diffusion through two basolateral chloride channels (CLC-Ka and CLC-Kb) (Figure 1.5). Both these channels must bind to a protein called barttin in order to be transported to the cell surface. A further chloride channel, CLC-5, is expressed at multiple sites in the nephron.

CALCIUM

Approximately 98% of filtered calcium is reabsorbed, 65 to 75% in the proximal tubule (via a paracellular pathway), 20 to 25% in the thick ascending limb of the loop of Henle, 10% in the distal tubule, and finally, small amounts in the collecting ducts. This is predominantly a passive process linked to active sodium reabsorption; for example, in the thick ascending limb of the loop of Henle, paracellular calcium transport is driven by the potential difference created by ROMK1. There are also active processes, particularly in the distal tubule, that tightly regulate the final amount of calcium excreted. Here, calcium reabsorption is transcellular and is predominantly under the control of parathyroid hormone (PTH) and the calcium-sensing receptor. Following entry into the cell from the lumen via an apical epithelial active transport mechanism (ECaC1), calcium binds to calbindin-D and is delivered to the basolateral membrane. Here it is extruded by a Ca^{2+}-ATPase (PMCA1b) and a sodium-calcium exchanger (NCX1). Transcription of both ECaC1 and calbindin is stimulated by calcitriol ($1,25(OH_2)D_3$), possibly synthesised locally in the distal nephron and acting in a paracrine and autocrine fashion. A functional vitamin D response element has been identified in the promotor region of the calbindin-D gene and there is a putative site in the ECaC1 gene. ECaC1 is a pH-sensitive, 83 kDa protein with six transmembrane spanning domains. Activation of the ion channel probably involves protein kinase C phosphorylation. There is evidence that stimulation of the renal calcium-sensing receptor can directly affect tubular reabsorption of calcium, independent of the effects of calciotropic hormones.

PHOSPHATE

Reabsorption of phosphate occurs predominantly in the proximal tubule and is mediated by a secondary active transport mechanism. Three families (types I, II and III) of sodium-dependent, phosphate cotransporters have been identified, of which type IIa, a 640 amino acid protein located in the apical plasma membrane, is thought to be the most physiologically important. Type IIa sodium/phosphate transport is electrogenic (i.e. involves the inward flux of a positive charge) with three sodium ions and one phosphate ion (preferentially divalent) being transferred. Acute regulation of transport is primarily achieved by an alteration in the amount of type IIa protein present in the apical membrane, with longer-term changes also involving increased transcription of the protein (e.g. in response to $1,25(OH_2)D_3$). Tonic levels of type IIa in the apical membrane are thought to be high, with regulation predominantly involving internalisation of the protein. Increased trafficking of the channel from the plasma membrane to the lysosomes is believed to follow both protein kinase A and C phosphorylation initiated by PTH receptor binding. Efflux of phosphate across the basolateral membrane may involve an anion exchange mechanism and/or a phosphate leak.

Normally less than 20% of the filtered load of phosphate is excreted into the urine, but above a plasma phosphate concentration of approximately 1.2 mmol/L increments in urinary phosphate excretion increase linearly with the filtered load, suggesting that there is T_m (tubular maximal uptake) for phosphate. The T_m for phosphate is influenced by the circulating PTH concentration and the ratio of T_m for phosphate to GFR (T_mP/GFR) has been used as a test in the differential diagnosis of hypercalcaemia. Although superseded in this context by modern PTH assays, it may still be useful in the investigation of inherited disorders of tubular phosphate handling.

BICARBONATE AND HYDROGEN ION

The kidney plays a central role in the maintenance of acid-base homeostasis through reclamation of filtered bicarbonate and excretion of acids through the titration of urinary buffers and excretion of ammonium. The former process predominantly takes place in the proximal tubule and the latter in the distal tubule. Disruption of these processes can cause renal tubular acidosis (see Chapter 5).

Proximal tubular bicarbonate reclamation is illustrated in Figure 1.7. Bicarbonate cannot be reabsorbed directly across the luminal membrane and has to be converted to carbon dioxide (CO_2) through a carbonic anhydrase mediated reaction; CO_2 can then diffuse into the tubular cells. The major processes involved are hydrogen ion secretion at the luminal (apical) membrane via a specific Na^+-H^+ exchanger (NHE-3) and bicarbonate transport at the basolateral membrane via a

Na^+-HCO_3^- cotransporter (NBC-1). Cytoplasmic carbonic anhydrase II (CA II) generates intracellular carbonic acid (H_2CO_3) and membrane-bound carbonic anhydrase IV (CA IV) catalyses the dissociation of luminal H_2CO_3. Approximately 80-90% of filtered bicarbonate is reabsorbed in the proximal tubule; the process is influenced by luminal and peritubular bicarbonate concentration, extracellular fluid volume, pCO_2, chloride, potassium, calcium, phosphate, PTH, glucocorticoids, α-adrenergic tone and AII. Both CA II and CA IV are stimulated under situations of metabolic acidosis.

Bicarbonate reabsorption in the proximal convoluted tubule

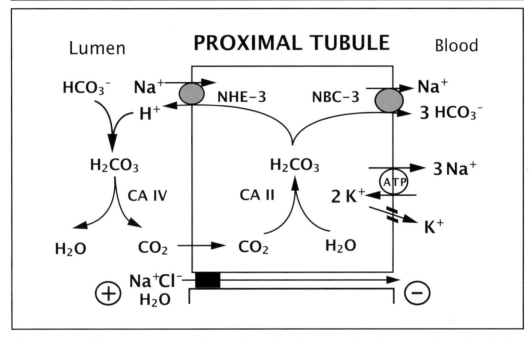

Figure 1.7 Bicarbonate reabsorption in the proximal convoluted tubule. Reproduced with permission from Soriano JR. Renal tubular acidosis: the clinical entity. J Am Soc Nephrol 2002; **13:** 2160-70.

Distal urinary acidification takes place by three mechanisms: (i) titration of divalent basic phosphate (HPO_4^{2-}) to form the monovalent acid form ($H_2PO_4^-$), (ii) accumulation of ammonia (NH_3) intraluminally which buffers hydrogen ion to form non-diffusible ammonium (NH_4^+), and (iii) reclamation of small amounts of bicarbonate that escape proximal tubular reabsorption. α-intercalated distal tubular cells are responsible for hydrogen ion secretion and β-intercalated cells for bicarbonate reclamation. Figure 1.8 illustrates the main processes in the α-intercalated cell. The main pump for luminal hydrogen ion secretion in the cell is a vacuolar H^+-ATPase. A H^+-K^+-ATPase is also involved in hydrogen ion secretion. Intracellularly formed bicarbonate leaves the cell via Cl^--HCO_3^- exchange, facilitated by an anion exchanger (AE1). Cytoplasmic CA II is necessary to secrete hydrogen ion. Acidification also occurs in the outer medullary collecting tubule against the electrochemical gradient via a vacuolar H^+-ATPase that is independent of sodium reabsorption. Distal acidification is influenced by blood pH and pCO_2, distal sodium transport, aldosterone and potassium.

Distal acidification in the cortical collecting tubule

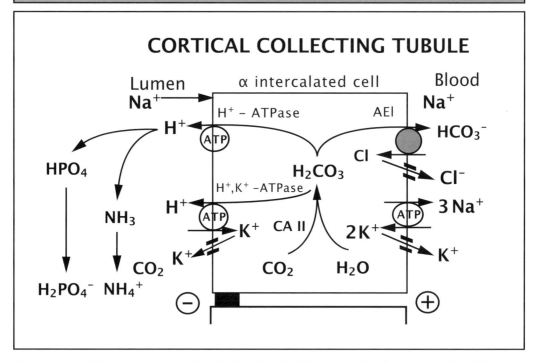

Figure 1.8 Schematic model of distal acidification in the cortical collecting tubule. Reproduced with permission from Soriano JR. Renal tubular acidosis: the clinical entity. J Am Soc Nephrol 2002; **13**: 2160-70.

Water homeostasis

The production of glomerular filtrate normally amounts to about 200 L/24 h. The unique physiology of the kidney enables approximately 99% of this to be reabsorbed in the production of urine with variable osmolality; between 50 and 1400 mosmol/kg at extremes of water intake. Plasma membranes of all mammalian cells are water permeable to variable degrees. In the kidney, different segments of the nephron show differing permeability to water, enabling the body to both retain water and produce urine of variable concentration. This process occurs both isosmotically, in association with electrolyte reabsorption in the proximal tubule, and differentially, in the loop of Henle, distal tubule and collecting duct in response to the action of the nonapeptide ADH. Absorption of water depends on the driving force for water reabsorption (predominantly active sodium transport) and the osmotic equilibration of water across the tubular epithelium. The generation of concentrated urine depends upon medullary hyperosmolality, which in turn requires low water permeability in some kidney segments (ascending limb of the loop of Henle), whereas in other kidney segments there is a requirement for high water permeability. Differing permeability and the facilitation of hormonal control is largely due to the differential expression along the nephron of a family of proteins known as the aquaporins, which act as water channels.

At least 11 different mammalian aquaporins (AQP) have now been recognised, of which seven (AQP1, -2, -3, -4, -6, -7, -8) are expressed in the kidney. Two asparagine-proline-alanine sequences in the molecule are thought to interact in the membrane to form a pathway for water translocation. AQP1 is found in the proximal tubule and descending thin limb of the loop of Henle and constitutes almost 3% of total membrane protein in the kidney. It appears to be constitutively expressed and is present in both the apical and basolateral plasma membranes, representing the entry and exit ports for water transport across the cell respectively. Approximately 70% of water reabsorption occurs at this site, predominantly via a transcellular (i.e. AQP1) rather than a paracellular route. Water reabsorption in the proximal tubule passively follows sodium reabsorption, so that the fluid entering the loop of Henle is still almost isosmotic with plasma.

Urinary concentration is predominantly achieved by countercurrent multiplication in the loop of Henle (Figure 1.9). Although the descending thin limb is very permeable to water, the ascending limb and the collecting duct are not (the collecting ducts are also poorly permeable to urea). The fluid entering the loop of Henle is isotonic to plasma but is hypotonic on leaving it. The ascending limb has active sodium reabsorption driven by Na^+-K^+-ATPase with electroneutralising transport of chloride, a combined process that can be inhibited by the so-called loop diuretics (e.g. furosemide). In this section of the nephron, sodium reabsorption is not accompanied by water, creating a hypertonic medullary interstitium and facilitating water reabsorption from the anatomically adjacent descending limb. The descending limb cells are permeable to sodium chloride, which is therefore cycled from the descending limb back to the ascending limb. The continuous flow along the loop generates an osmotic gradient at the tip of the loop that can reach 1400 mosmol/kg. Approximately 5% of water is reabsorbed in the loop of Henle.

Countercurrent multiplication mechanism

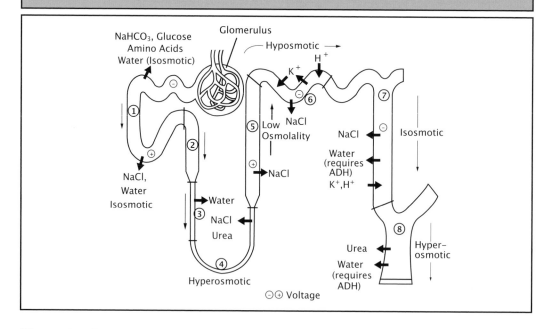

Figure 1.9 Countercurrent multiplication mechanism: schematic representation of the principal processes of transport in the nephron. In the convoluted portion of the proximal tubule (1), salts and water are reabsorbed at high rates in isotonic proportions. Bulk reabsorption of most of the filtrate (65-70%) and virtually complete reabsorption of glucose, amino acids, and bicarbonate take place in this segment. In the pars recta (2), organic acids are secreted and continuous reabsorption of sodium chloride takes place. The loop of Henle comprises three segments: the thin descending (3) and ascending (4) limbs and the thick ascending limb (5). The fluid becomes hyperosmotic, because of water abstraction, as it flows toward the bend of the loop, and hyposmotic, because of sodium chloride reabsorption, as it flows toward the distal convoluted tubule (6). Active sodium reabsorption occurs in the distal convoluted tubule and in the cortical collecting tubule (7). This latter segment is water-impermeable in the absence of ADH and the reabsorption of sodium in this segment is increased by aldosterone. The collecting duct (8) allows equilibration of water with the hyperosmotic interstitium when ADH is present. For further details, see text. Reproduced with permission from Burg MB: The nephron in transport of sodium, amino acids, and glucose. Hospital Practice 1978; **13**: 100.

A further 10% of water reabsorption occurs in the distal tubule, with the remainder (more than 20 L/24 h) being reabsorbed in the collecting ducts. Entry of water into the collecting duct cells occurs via apical AQP2 channels with exit probably occurring via basolateral AQP3 (cortical and outer medullary collecting ducts) and AQP4 (inner medullary collecting ducts). AQP2 appears to be the primary target for ADH regulation of water reabsorption. AQP2 is stored in sub-apical vesicles in the collecting duct cells. In response to ADH stimulation these vesicles are cycled, and inserted into the plasma membrane by a cytoskeletal, dynein-mediated, transport process. ADH stimulation occurs following binding of ADH to a V_2 receptor in the plasma membrane, which stimulates a cAMP/protein kinase A cascade resulting in phosphorylation and activation of AQP2. ADH regulates the acute cellular water-retaining response (AQP2 trafficking) and also its longer-term regulation, via a conditioning effect on AQP2 gene transcription. It is likely that there are also ADH-independent regulatory pathways of AQP2 expression. Membrane insertion of AQP2 allows water to pass into the collecting duct cells under the influence of medullary hyperosmolality. Maintenance of medullary hyperosmolality also depends upon efficient fluid removal, which is the function of the ascending vasa recta, a specialized medullary vasculature, and the close anatomical relations of all the medullary constituents (Figure 1.2). AQP2 expression is decreased in a variety of polyuric conditions (e.g. diabetes insipidus, lithium treatment, hypokalaemia, hypercalcaemia, urinary obstruction) and increased in some-water retaining states (e.g. heart failure, pregnancy).

ADH also increases the permeability of collecting duct cells to urea, which is the major osmotically active component of the luminal fluid in the distal tubule. Fluid of high urea concentration therefore enters the deepest layers of the medullary interstitium, passing down its concentration gradient, contributing to medullary hyperosmolality. The regulation of ADH secretion is of vital importance to fluid homeostasis. The normal plasma osmolality is maintained very tightly between 280 and 295 mmol/kg and is regulated by means of specific osmoreceptors found in the anterior hypothalamus. These receptors modulate the release of ADH and also affect thirst. ADH release can also be stimulated by hypotension, hypovolaemia and vomiting, independently of osmoregulation.

Endocrine function
The endocrine functions of the kidneys may be regarded both as primary, because the kidneys are endocrine organs producing hormones, and as secondary, because the kidneys are a site of action for hormones produced or activated elsewhere. In addition, the kidneys are a site of degradation for hormones such as insulin and aldosterone. In their primary endocrine function, the kidneys produce EPO, renin, prostaglandins and $1,25(OH_2)D_3$.

The biology of EPO and the use of recombinant human erythropoietin (rhEPO, Epoetin) in the management of anaemia of kidney disease is discussed in Chapter

6. Prostaglandins and thromboxanes are synthesised from arachidonic acid by the cyclooxygenase enzyme system. This system is present in many parts of the kidney and has an important role in regulating the physiological action of other hormones on renal vascular tone, mesangial contractility and tubular processing of salt and water. In pathophysiological circumstances, such as acute glomerulonephritis and various forms of acute renal failure, thromboxane A_2 and various prostaglandins may have a significant role in inflammation and alteration of vascular tone. The importance of renin in the maintenance of systemic blood pressure is discussed above (see Juxtaglomerular Apparatus). The kidneys are primarily responsible for producing $1,25(OH_2)D_3$ from 25-hydroxycholecalciferol as a result of the action of the enzyme 25-hydroxycholecalciferol 1α-hydroxylase found in proximal tubular epithelial cells. The regulation of this system and its disturbance in kidney disease is considered in Chapter 6.

Glomerular filtration rate (GFR)

The GFR is considered to be the most reliable measure of the functional capacity of the kidneys and is often thought of as indicative of the number of functioning nephrons. As a physiological measurement it has proved to be the most sensitive and specific marker of changes in overall renal function (see Chapter 3).

The rate of formation of the glomerular filtrate depends upon the balance between hydrostatic and oncotic forces along the afferent arteriole and across the glomerular filter. The maintenance of renal blood flow is essential to kidney function and there is a complex array of intrarenal regulatory mechanisms ensuring that the renal glomerular perfusion pressure is maintained at a constant 45 mm Hg across a wide range of systemic blood pressures. These mechanisms include modulators of vascular tone (e.g. nitric oxide, AII, prostaglandins, ANP and adenosine) and the renal sympathetic nervous system. The net pressure difference across the glomerular filtration barrier must be sufficient not only to drive filtration, but also to drive the ultrafiltrate along the tubules against their inherent resistance to flow. In the absence of sufficient pressure, the lumina of the tubules will collapse.

Glomerular permeability and protein handling

The glomerulus acts as a selective filter of the blood passing through its capillaries. The combination of a specialised endothelium, epithelial cell barrier, and basement membrane rich in negatively charged proteoglycans produces a fibre-matrix filter that restricts the passage of macromolecules in a size, charge and shape dependent manner (Figure 1.3). The fibres are separated by interstices about 2 nm wide, but the basement membrane is a compressible filter, becoming more permeable as the applied pressure decreases and the fibres separate.

The glomerular permeability of a molecule is expressed in terms of its glomerular sieving coefficient (GSC). Molecules smaller than approximately the molecular weight of inulin (5 kDa) are freely filtered. Therefore, inulin, urea, creatinine, glucose and electrolytes all have a GSC = 1.0. Classic experiments have used linear dextran chains of varying molecular weight and charge to study glomerular filtration characteristics. However, linear carbohydrate chains do not necessarily behave in the same manner as a globular protein of equal molecular weight or charge. For example, neutral dextran chains of 15 kDa (diameter 2.4 nm) have GSC = 1.0 whereas β2-microglobulin (11.8 kDa, diameter 1.6 nm) has GSC = 0.7. Figure 1.10 gives examples of the relationships between size, charge and mass of the major urinary proteins and their glomerular handling.

The protein concentration in the glomerular filtrate has been measured in a number of animal models by direct glomerular puncture. The concentration of total protein found is in the range of several hundred mg/L (approximately 1% of that of plasma), with albumin concentrations ranging from a few hundred to less than 40 mg/L. The filtered load of protein depends on the product of the GSC and the free plasma concentration; therefore the albumin load per nephron is much greater than that of the other filtered proteins. In general, proteins of molecular weight greater than albumin (66 kDa, diameter 3.5 nm) are retained by the healthy glomerulus and are termed high molecular weight proteins.

The urinary concentration of proteins depends upon the filtered load and on the efficiency of the proximal tubular reabsorptive process. Proteins are reabsorbed by receptor-mediated, low-affinity, high-capacity procesess. Recently, the importance of two endocytic, multi-ligand receptors, megalin (600 kDa) and cubulin (460 kDa), in protein reabsorption has been recognised. Megalin belongs to the LDL-receptor family whereas cubulin is identical to the intestinal intrinsic factor-vitamin B_{12} receptor. In the kidney, both are localised in clathrin-coated pits in the apical brush border of renal proximal tubular cells and bind filtered proteins in a calcium-dependent process. Megalin appears capable of both binding and internalising its ligands whereas the cubulin-ligand complex requires megalin to be internalised. Some proteins (e.g. albumin) can bind to either receptor, whereas others are specific (e.g. transferrin binds to cubilin only and retinol binding protein (RBP) and α_1-microglobulin to megalin only). Once proteins have been internalised, they are transported by the endocytic vesicle and fuse with lysosomes. Proteolysis occurs and the resultant amino acids are released into the tubulo-interstitial space across the basolateral surface of the tubular epithelial cell. The membrane vesicles are then recycled to the brush border to complete the reabsorption cycle by returning the receptors. In health, the reabsorptive mechanism removes 99% of the filtered protein, thus retaining most of their essential amino acid constituents for re-use. Capture of filtered transport proteins is important in conserving vitamin status (e.g. vitamin A associated with RBP). Tubular secretion of proteins also contributes to urinary total protein concentration; in particular, Tamm-Horsfall glycoprotein (THG), accounts for ~50% of urinary total protein. The normal urinary total protein excretion is less than 150 mg/24 h.

Major urinary proteins

Protein	Mr (kDa)	Free plasma conc. (g/L)	Diameter (nm)	pI	Glomerular sieving coefficient	Filtered load (mg/L)[a]	Urinary conc. (mg/L)
IgG	150	10	5.5	7.3	0.0001	1	0.1
Albumin	66	40	3.5	4.7	0.0002	8	5
α1-microglobulin	31	0.025	2.9	4.5	~0.3	7.5	5
Retinol binding protein	22	0.025	2.1	4.5	~0.7	17.5	0.1
Cystatin C	12.8	0.01	?	9.2	~0.7	0.7	0.1
β2-microglobulin	11.8	0.015	1.6	5.6	0.7	1.1	0.1

[a]concentration in the glomerular filtrate

Figure 1.10 Characteristics of some major urinary proteins.

Changes to kidney function during life

Kidney function is not constant throughout life. *In utero*, urine is produced by the developing fetus from about the ninth week of gestation. Nephrogenesis is complete by approximately 35 weeks gestation, although kidney function remains immature during the first two years of life. The kidneys of the term infant receive approximately 6% of the cardiac output, compared to 25% in adults. Renal vascular resistance is relatively high and the low renal blood flow is particularly directed to the medulla and inner cortex. The gradual increase in renal blood flow that occurs with increasing age is mainly directed to the outer cortex and is mediated by local neurohormonal mechanisms. The GFR at birth is approximately 30 mL/min/1.73 m^2. It increases rapidly during the first weeks of life to reach approximately 70 mL/min/1.73 m^2 by 16 days of age. Normal adult values are achieved by 14 years of age. Tubular function, including salt and water conservation, is also immature at birth. Birth is associated with rapid changes in kidney function, with a switch to salt and water conservation being mediated by catecholamines, the renin-angiotensin system, vasopressin, glucocorticoids and thyroid hormone. The immaturity of the neonatal kidney contributes to the relatively common problems of water and electrolyte disturbances in infants. It follows that these are more likely to occur in premature infants, particularly those born before 35 weeks gestation.

Older age is associated with a range of structural changes in the kidney, including decreasing weight, total renal area, cortical area and number of glomeruli. The percentage of sclerotic glomeruli increases, particularly in the cortical zone. These changes are paralleled by changes in the afferent and efferent arteriolar systems, with sclerosis of the cortical systems and the formation of direct channels (shunts) between the afferent and efferent arterioles in the medulla. Ageing is also associated with the development of tubulointerstitial fibrosis, loss of tubular mass and decreasing length of the proximal tubule.

Structural change is accompanied by functional changes, which in many respects are the reverse of those seen in early life. On average, GFR declines with age by approximately 1 mL/min/1.73 m^2/y over the age of 40 years of age and the rate of decline in GFR accelerates after the age of 65 years. Renal blood flow also decreases with age, whilst the filtration fraction (i.e. GFR/renal plasma flow) and renal vascular resistance increase. Blood flow to the renal cortex would appear to be particularly affected. The higher filtration fraction of the deeper juxtamedullary glomeruli may, in part, explain the increase in filtration fraction with ageing; this may be an adaptive response to structural change helping to preserve kidney function in the ageing individual. Tubular function (ability to concentrate urine and excrete a water and salt load) is decreased and nocturnal polyuria is common. Renal salt conservation is also impaired and urinary albumin excretion increases with age. It is not known whether these changes are the result of a normal ageing process (i.e. involutional) or the result of the interplay of pathology and age.

Further reading

GENERAL ANATOMY AND PHYSIOLOGY
Brenner BM. Brenner and Rector's The Kidney, 7th edition, Saunders, Philadelphia, 2004.

Lote C. Principles of Renal Physiology, 4th edition, Kluwer Academic Publishers, Dordrecht, Boston, London, 2000.

ELECTROLYTE HOMEOSTASIS
Greger R. Why do loop diuretics cause hypokalaemia? Nephrol Dial Transplant 1997; **12:** 1799-801.

AQUAPORINS
Nielsen S, Kwon TH, Christensen BM, Promeneur D, Frokiaer J, Marples D. Physiology and pathophysiology of renal aquaporins. J Am Soc Nephrol 1999; **10:** 647-63.

Nielsen S, Frokiaer J, Marples D, Kwon TH, Agre P, Knepper MA. Aquaporins in the kidney: from molecules to medicine. Physiol Rev 2002; **82:** 205-44.

PROTEIN HANDLING
Verroust PJ, Christensen EI. Megalin and cubilin—the story of two multipurpose receptors unfolds. Nephrol Dial Transplant 2002; **17:** 1867-71.

AGEING AND THE KIDNEY
Epstein M. Aging and the kidney. J Am Soc Nephrol 1996; **7:** 1106-22.

Lamb EJ, O'Riordan SE, Delaney MP. Ageing and the kidney: pathology, assessment and management. Clin Chim Acta 2003; **334:** 25-40.

Chapter 2

Kidney disease: an introduction and overview

Introduction

The global burden of kidney disease is increasing rapidly. Kidney disease is now recognised as a public health problem with ever increasing economic costs and poor clinical outcome. Although the incidence and prevalence of patients requiring renal replacement therapy (RRT) has increased over the last three decades, it is now apparent that advanced kidney disease is only the tip of a very large iceberg. Recent data from the Third National Health and Nutrition Examination Survey (NHANES III) estimated that 11% (19.2 million) of the adult population in the United States (US) suffers from chronic kidney disease (CKD), with 4.7% (8.3 million) in CKD stages 3-5. In contrast, the United States Renal Data System (USRDS), a vast national database of patients receiving RRT, reports an estimated prevalence of end-stage renal disease (ESRD) in the US population of 344,000. It appears, therefore, that only a small percentage of the CKD population progresses to RRT. Similar data have been obtained from populations in the United Kingdom (UK) and Australia. The prevalence of CKD is much higher in older age groups and especially in people with diabetes mellitus and hypertension. Many patients with documented kidney disease are unknown to nephrology services. A study from east Kent in the UK using the laboratory database identified a prevalence of CKD of 5.5%. Of this cohort only 15% were known to the nephrology centre. The non-referred group were elderly, with a median age of 83 years. Defining and screening the populations at risk of progressive kidney disease is now one of the major challenges facing both nephrology and the wider medical community.

Treatment of advanced kidney disease is expensive and RRT is increasingly utilised in a broad range of patients with CKD. In many cases patients are elderly and have substantial co-morbidity associated with cardiovascular disease and diabetes (Figure 2.1). In the UK, between 2 and 3% of the National Health Service (NHS) budget is spent on dialysis and transplantation. In the US, spending on ESRD during 2002 was in excess of $20 billion, with growth in this area of greater than 100% in the past ten years. This is forecast to increase by another 75% within the next ten years.

Renal disease in the US

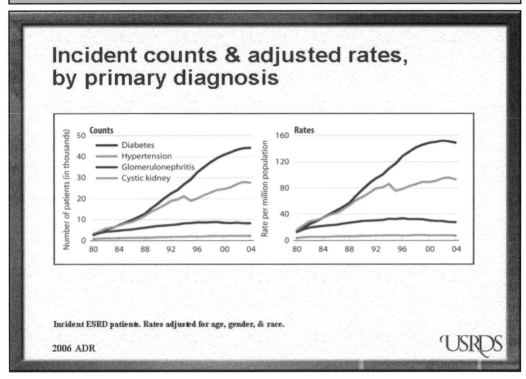

Incident counts & adjusted rates, by primary diagnosis

Incident ESRD patients. Rates adjusted for age, gender, & race.

2006 ADR

'USRDS

Figure 2.1 Incident counts by primary diagnosis and adjusted rates by primary diagnosis in the United States. The number of new patients taken onto dialysis programmes has increased over the past 15 years or so. In the US much of this increase is a result of diabetes-related kidney disease. The incidence of glomerulonephritis as the cause of end-stage kidney disease remains constant. The right hand panel shows that the incident rate of new patients to dialysis with a primary diagnosis of diabetes is almost 160 per million population. To place this in context with UK practice, this is in excess of the incident rate for all diagnoses of 108 per million population in 2005 in the UK (data not shown).

US Renal Data System: Excerpts from the USRDS 2006 Annual Data Report. Am J Kidney Dis 49:S1-S296 (suppl 1). The data reported here have been supplied by the United States Renal Data System (USRDS). The interpretation and reporting of these data are the responsibility of the authors and in no way should be seen as an official policy or interpretation of the US government.

Chronic kidney disease

Definition and classification

Given the high cost and relatively poor outcomes of RRT in terms of patient survival on dialysis, a number of organisations have developed guidelines and standards for investigation and treatment. For example, the UK Renal Association published the first edition of a standards document in 1995 and subsequent editions have built on this. In the US, the National Kidney Foundation's Kidney Disease Outcomes Quality Initiative (K/DOQI) Clinical Practice Guidelines on CKD were published in 2002 and have provided the basis for current recommendations for classification and treatment of CKD (Figure 2.2). The older term of chronic renal failure (CRF) has largely been abandoned and CKD is the preferred nomenclature. Kidney failure is defined as either (1) a GFR < 15 mL/min/1.73 m^2, which is accompanied in most cases by signs and symptoms of uraemia, or (2) a need for initiation of RRT (dialysis or transplantation) to treat the complications of decreased GFR, which would otherwise increase the risk of mortality and morbidity. Some patients may need dialysis or transplantation at GFR ≥ 15 mL/min/1.73 m^2 because of symptoms of uraemia. The K/DOQI Work Group acknowledged that the level of GFR selected for this definition is arbitrary and may need to be modified based on advances in RRT.

ESRD is an administrative term in the US, based on the conditions for payment for health care by the Medicare ESRD Program, specifically the level of GFR and the occurrence of signs and symptoms of kidney failure necessitating initiation of treatment by RRT. ESRD includes patients treated by dialysis or transplantation, irrespective of the level of GFR. The K/DOQI definition of kidney failure differs in two important ways from this definition of ESRD. Firstly, not all individuals with GFR < 15 mL/min/1.73 m^2 or with signs and symptoms of kidney failure are treated by dialysis or transplantation. Nonetheless, such individuals should be considered as having kidney failure. Secondly, among treated patients, kidney transplant recipients have a higher mean GFR (usually 30 to 60 mL/min/1.73 m^2) following transplantation and better average health outcomes than dialysis patients. Kidney transplant recipients should not be included in the definition of kidney failure unless they have a GFR < 15 mL/min/1.73 m^2 or have resumed dialysis. In the UK, the National Service Framework (NSF) for Renal Services refers to CKD that has progressed such that RRT is required to maintain life as 'established renal failure' (ERF; sometimes called end-stage renal failure, ESRF).

International classification of CKD

Stage	Description	GFR mL/min/ 1.73 m²	Population prevalence (%)	Metabolic consequences	Management
1[a]	Kidney damage with normal or increased GFR	> 90	3.3	Hypertension more frequent than amongst patients without CKD.	Treatment of comorbid conditions. Slowing progression. CVD risk reduction.
2[a]	Kidney damage with mildly decreasing GFR	60-89	3.0	Hypertension frequent. Concentration of parathyroid hormone (PTH) starts to rise (GFR 60-80).	Estimating progression.
3[b]	Moderately decreased GFR	30-59	4.3	Hypertension frequent. Decrease in calcium absorption (GFR < 50). Increased PTH concentration. Reduced phosphate excretion. Malnutrition. Left ventricular hypertrophy. anaemia (erythropoietin deficiency).	Evaluating and treating complications.
4	Severely reduced GFR	15-29	0.2	As above but more pronounced, plus: triglyceride concentrations start to rise; metabolic acidosis; decreased libido; hyperphosphataemia; tendency to hyperkalaemia.	Preparation for RRT (creation of dialysis access, assessment for potential transplantation).
5	Kidney failure (established renal failure[c])	< 15	0.2	As above but more pronounced plus: saline retention causing apparent heart failure; anorexia; vomiting; pruritis (without skin disease).	RRT, if uraemia present.

[a]The diagnosis of stage 1 and 2 CKD requires the presence of kidney damage for ≥ 3 months manifest by pathological abnormalities of the kidney or abnormalities in the composition of urine, such as haematuria or proteinuria, or abnormalities in imaging tests either with (stage 2) or without (stage 1), decreases in GFR.

[b]Recent guidelines from the National Institute for Health and Clinical Excellence (NICE) have suggested subdivision of Stage 3 into 3a (GFR 45-59 mL/min/1.73m²) and 3b (GFR 30-44 mL/min/1.73m²).

[c]In the National Service Framework for Renal Services, the term 'kidney failure' in the National Kidney Foundation classification has been replaced by 'established renal failure' (ERF) defined as 'chronic kidney disease which has progressed so far that renal replacement therapy is needed to maintain life'.

CVD = cardiovascular disease, GFR = glomerular filtration rate, RRT = renal replacement therapy.

Figure 2.2. The international classification of CKD indicating metabolic and management consequences. Prevalence data are based upon the NHANES III survey of a North American population.

The K/DOQI guidelines have been widely distributed and are welcomed as they will facilitate performance of comparative studies and analysis. Criteria for the definition of CKD are:

1) **Kidney damage** for ≥ 3 months, as defined by structural or functional abnormalities of the kidney, with or without decreased GFR, which can lead to decreased GFR, manifest by either: (a) pathological abnormalities, or (b) markers of kidney damage, including abnormalities in the composition of the blood or urine, or abnormalities in imaging tests.

2) **GFR < 60 mL/min/1.73 m^2** for ≥ 3 months, with or without kidney damage.

Kidney 'damage' in many diseases can be ascertained by the presence of proteinuria/albuminuria. In turn, GFR can be estimated from equations based on the serum creatinine concentration. The assessment of kidney function is explored in detail in Chapter 3. However, the rationale for the use of the cut-off of < 60 mL/min/1.73 m^2 is worthy of note here. Although, it is now increasingly recognised that complications of CKD may develop with this degree of glomerular dysfunction, crucially there is an increased risk of cardiovascular disease and death associated with moderate kidney disease. CKD has been demonstrated to be an independent risk factor for cardiovascular death and many more individuals die as a result of cardiovascular disease than progress to advanced kidney disease. Importantly, CKD is now recognised as a risk factor for cardiovascular disease and therefore detection of CKD alerts the physician to the need to modify other relevant risk factors.

The criteria for diagnosis of CKD as above do not include the cause of the CKD. Once the presence of CKD is established according to the listed criteria it is important to *classify* based on the level of function. The present classification system is based on glomerular function. However, other factors, including degree of proteinuria and cause of kidney disease, influence prognosis; further research is necessary to devise a classification system that takes these prognostic factors into consideration. Complications typical of CKD can be investigated and treated (see Chapter 6) and clinical guidelines for management of patients with CKD have been established (see Chapter 8). A rapid deterioration in kidney function is referred to as acute renal failure (ARF) and this is discussed in Chapter 4.

Ethnicity and epidemiology
Worldwide epidemiological evidence indicates that the incidence of CKD is increased in many ethnic minorities. In the UK, the incidence of CKD and RRT are 3-5 times greater in Asian and African-Caribbean populations than in a comparable Caucasian population. The increased risk is largely due to the increased

prevalence of diabetes and hypertension in these populations. The USRDS esti-mates the lifetime risk of developing ESRD in 20 year old black men and women respectively to be 7.3% and 7.8%, compared to 2.5% in white men and 1.8% in white women. Family history of kidney disease is a risk factor for developing ESRD in both white and black Americans, but particularly among blacks in the US there is a nine-fold increased risk for ESRD among those individuals with a first-degree relative with ESRD. There may therefore be genetic influences for the development of kidney disease and for the rate of progression to ESRD. In more homogeneous populations the increased incidence of ESRD is even more marked. Members of the native American Pima tribe are very susceptible to diabetic nephropathy. Another example is the Aboriginal population in Tiwi Island, Northern Territory, Australia, in which obesity and type 2 diabetes are endemic and the ESRD incidence exceeds 2000/million population/year. This population has been the target of improved health promotion and early intervention to treat diabetes and hypertension and there is evidence of more favorable outcomes.

The pattern of diseases that are causing the increased incidence and prevalence of ESRD are changing and vary between nation states. For example, diabetes is the cause of ESRD in approximately 40% of new patients in the US, but only 20% of new patients in the UK. Hypertension is particularly prevalent in the US as the cause of ESRD among black and Asian patients. Other diseases such as glomeru-lonephritis, polycystic kidneys and renovascular disease make up the majority of other causes; 25% of cases were recorded as 'aetiology uncertain' in the UK in 2003 according to the UK Renal Registry, illustrating the difficulties of accurate diagnosis. Kidney failure is common in developing countries, with socioeconomic and local environmental factors determining the pattern of disease. For example, human immunodeficiency virus (HIV) infection in sub-Saharan Africa can cause kidney failure and is an ever increasing problem. Other forms of glomeru-lonephritis are related to endemic infections such as malaria and hepatitis B. However, diabetes is emerging as a major epidemic in the developing world and will contribute significantly to CKD in these populations.

Diagnosing kidney disease

Clinical presentation
The clinical presentation of kidney disease is highly variable (Figure 2.3). The majority of kidney disease is detected opportunistically by measurement of blood pressure, urine testing and blood tests in asymptomatic individuals. This can occur in the primary care setting or for health clearance purposes for insurance. Typical findings include isolated haematuria and isolated proteinuria. Kidney disease may also present with macroscopic haematuria, swollen ankles,

headaches and visual disturbances due to severe hypertension, or as a manifestation of systemic disease such as in the vasculitides and systemic lupus erythematosus (SLE).

Symptoms of kidney disease

Symptoms of CKD	Signs of CKD	Investigations	Comments
Incidental finding	None	Urine dipstick confirms microscopic haematuria and/or proteinuria	Insurance or occupational medical
Screening populations at risk of CKD e.g. hypertension, cardiovascular disease, diabetes, obesity, family history	Hypertension and evidence of end-organ damage, vascular disease, diabetic retinopathy	Screen for proteinuria and estimate GFR	Consider atheromatous renal artery stenosis particularly if GFR falls by 20% on introduction of RAAS blockade
Macroscopic haematuria	Painless or painful. Associated features may include weight loss, fever, pain on passing urine	Urine testing, GFR, exclude infection. Imaging of renal tract to include kidneys, ureters and bladder. Cystoscopy. Kidney biopsy	May present to urologist. Consider kidney stones and urinary tract infection. Renal cell carcinoma, ureteric and bladder tumours. IgA nephropathy, Alport's syndrome in association with proteinuria
Smoky urine and swollen legs and eyes	May follow streptococcal infection Oedematous legs	Urine testing confirming haematuria and heavy proteinuria. Decline in GFR	Likely glomerulonephritis. Wide differential diagnosis. Renal biopsy indicated in adults where diagnosis uncertain
Very swollen legs Frothy urine		Nephrotic range proteinuria, hypoalbuminuria, absent or minimal haematuria	Nephrotic syndrome
Lethargy, poor appetite and vomiting	Pallor, sallow complexion, excoriations, fluid retention, audible pericardial rub, confusion	Investigate for advanced CKD. Consider secondary causes	Advanced kidney disease. Arrange RRT or conservative management
Poor urine stream, increased frequency of micturition	Palpable bladder. In male patients a digital rectal examination may detect prostate abnormalities	Ultrasound scan of kidneys and bladder. Trial of urinary catheterisation	Obstructive uropathy/ bladder outflow obstruction

RAAS = renin-angiotensin-aldosterone system

Figure 2.3 Typical presenting symptoms and signs of kidney disease.

Symptoms suggestive of advanced kidney disease (i.e. patients with stage 4 and stage 5 CKD) include fatigue, nausea, vomiting, poor appetite, shortness of breath, fluid retention, poor memory, loss of libido and itching. These patients are often very ill and malnourished and are considered for RRT. Unfortunately, as many as 30% of individuals present very late in their disease and may require urgent dialysis without having been previously known to the specialist nephrology service. These patients have been shown to have a poor prognosis compared to patients that have been cared for in a multidisciplinary specialist environment for at least one year. Therefore, early recognition of kidney disease is of paramount importance to outcome.

Diagnosis of kidney disease requires a detailed history to include current symptoms, past medical and family history, social history and a full drug history. A focused examination may identify potential causes of kidney disease such as obstructive uropathy or may indicate vascular disease associated with narrowing of the arteries supplying the kidneys (atheromatous renal artery stenosis (ARAS)), systemic disease or *de novo* kidney disease. The blood pressure and dipstick examination of the urine (urinalysis) are crucial baseline assessments.

Imaging of the urinary tract
Imaging of the renal tract to include kidneys, ureters, bladder and prostate gland is very important in many kidney diseases and provides useful information. It is mandatory in all cases of new ARF to identify size, symmetry of kidneys and to exclude obstruction to urine flow anywhere within the tract. Renal ultrasound is the imaging technique of choice in the majority of cases and gives reliable data on size of kidneys and evidence of obstruction where present (Figure 2.4). Additionally, underlying structural abnormalities such as polycystic kidneys, renal cysts and tumours and anatomical and congenital malformations may be demonstrated. Renal ultrasonography is simple, cheap, non-invasive and without risk. Intravenous urography/pyelography (IVU/IVP) is utilised mainly in urological practice to identify kidney stone disease and to investigate structural disease of the urinary tract such as a transitional cell carcinoma of the ureter or bladder. Diagnostic IVU may be difficult to perform in renal impairment. The incidence of allergic reactions to the contrast medium is low using modern non-ionic contrast media. Imaging of soft tissues with either computed tomography (CT) scanning or magnetic resonance imaging (MRI) may also be necessary to identify structural abnormalities. CT has a role in the investigation of acute loin pain and is particularly helpful in the detection of ureteric calculi.

Invasive investigations of the urinary tract, particularly in obstruction and haematuria, include a cystoscopic examination of the bladder lining under direct vision. This also allows for selective cannulation of each ureteric orifice and imaging with X-rays following injection of radiocontrast medium (retrograde study). The level of the lesion in an obstructed kidney can also be ascertained by percutaneous insertion of a catheter into the kidney via a nephrostomy and subsequent injection of contrast via the nephrostomy tube with X-rays taken as the contrast is drained from the kidney into the ureter and bladder (antegrade study).

Ultrasound scan of a kidney

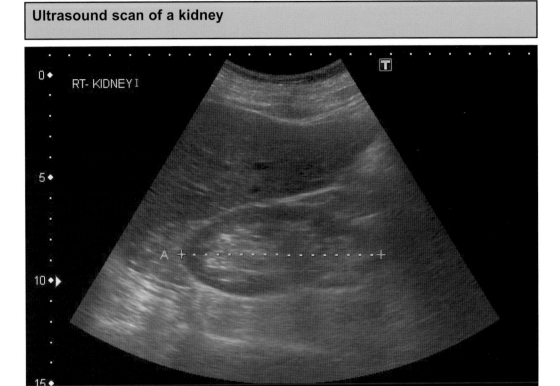

Figure 2.4 Ultrasound scan of a kidney in longitudinal section. The renal pelvis is non-dilated and the cortex is readily identifiable. A biopsy is taken from the lower pole away from the hilar vessels. The homogeneous mass that can be seen above the kidney is the liver.

Nuclear medicine scintigraphy is used to identify scars or cortical defects within kidneys and to assess the differential function of each kidney relative to the other. Static renal scanning uses technetium-^{99m}-dimercaptosuccinic acid (^{99m}Tc-DMSA), which binds to proximal renal tubules. Three hours after injection of the isotope the kidneys are imaged. The scan can define the differential function of each kidney and identifies scarring. Dynamic renography uses radiolabelled tracers that are excreted rapidly by the kidneys. Images are obtained by gamma camera. Commonly used tracers are ^{99m}Tc-diethylenetriaminepentaacetic acid

(^{99m}Tc-DTPA) and ^{99m}Tc-mercaptoacetyltriglycerine (^{99m}Tc-MAG3). Patients with well preserved kidney function that are suspected of having renal artery stenosis may be challenged with an ACE inhibitor, such as captopril and dynamic renograms obtained to assess whether the flow of the radioisotope alters significantly following captopril administration. Radioisotopes are also utilised in some cases when obstruction is suspected, but cannot be reliably demonstrated on ultrasound scanning or when the collecting system within the kidney is dilated, to assess whether there is a functional obstruction. The excretion of the radioisotope is tested following the administration of a loop diuretic.

Further investigation for suspected ARAS can be performed by selective renal angiography. This can be achieved following X-ray screening of a fine bore catheter inserted into the aorta via the femoral artery (most commonly) or brachial artery. Magnetic resonance angiography (MRA) is proving a valuable tool in the non-invasive testing of patients for renovascular disease such as ARAS. The image quality is now excellent and MRA is likely to supersede selective renal angiography for diagnosis of renovascular disease. The renal arteries can be studied following injection with gadolinium contrast medium (Figures 2.5 (a) and (b)). Following selective renal angiography, angioplasty and stent deployment, the patency of the vessel can be improved (Figure 2.6).

Magnetic resonance angiogram (MRA) of renal blood vessels

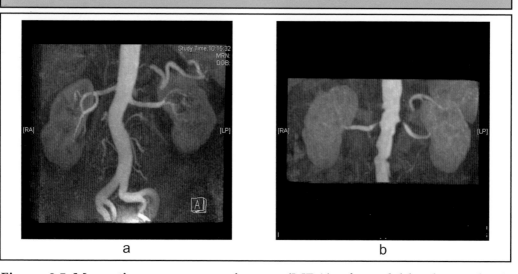

a

b

Figure 2.5 Magnetic resonance angiogram (MRA) of renal blood vessels. A normal angiogram (a) demonstrates no evidence of narrowing to pristine renal arteries. In contrast, bilateral renal artery stenosis is demonstrated (b) with narrowing to the arterial lumen at the ostial opening to the aorta.

Kidney stent

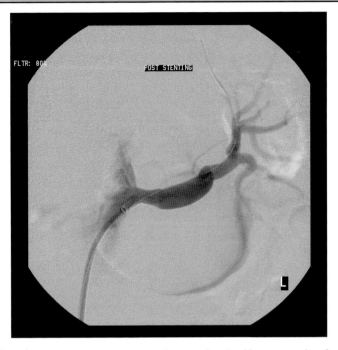

Figure 2.6 Following percutaneous angiography, balloon angioplasty and radiological deployment of a metal stent within the renal artery, the vessel patency is dramatically improved.

Kidney biopsy

Renal biopsies are performed by specialist nephrologists and renal transplant surgeons to investigate kidney disease in highly selected cases. It is essential that an experienced pathologist familiar with kidney diseases examines the specimen. A biopsy is helpful in unexplained renal failure, nephrotic syndrome, moderate proteinuria and haematuria and in a failing kidney transplant. A biopsy specimen is taken from only one kidney and is generally performed using local anaesthetic. In an effort to reduce the risk of haemorrhage, the specimen is taken from the lower pole of the kidney away from the hilum, after checking that coagulation and platelet function are normal. Anti-platelet drugs such as aspirin should be discontinued where possible. The lower pole is identified using ultrasound scanning and a semi-automatic needle device is placed on the capsule of the kidney and released into the cortex and medulla. A sample of tissue is obtained for light microscopy (LM), immunofluorescence or immunoperoxidase (IM) staining as well as electron microscopy (EM). It should be emphasised that although approximately 11% of the adult population may have CKD, only a tiny minority of patients undergo a kidney biopsy. Few patients with ARF undergo renal biopsy since the cause of ARF is usually clinically evident (see Chapter 4). Biopsy of suspected renal malignancy is undertaken following collaboration with urologists and radiologists and need not necessarily be referred to the nephrologist.

The kidney biopsy findings provide some indication of the prognosis of kidney disease. Data from a large series of patients have correlated the degree of tubulointerstitial fibrosis and scarring with outcome in CKD. However, it must be remembered that the biopsy is a tiny sample of kidney and may or may not represent the entire kidney architecture. However, even in proteinuric kidney disease, damage to the tubulointerstitial compartment has greater prognostic index than the degree of glomerular damage. Recent hypotheses have suggested that glomerular damage with subsequent proteinuria stimulates a myriad of inflammatory changes within the tubules and tubulointerstitial space resulting in tipping the balance from healing to scarring. Much of this pro-inflammatory milieu is generated directly or indirectly by AII and aldosterone-dependent mechanisms and this may explain some of the contribution of drugs such as ACE inhibitors and angiotensin receptor blockers (ARBs) in protecting kidney function over and above their effect on blood pressure.

Progression of chronic kidney disease

Pathophysiology of CKD progression

The kidneys have considerable reserve capacity to increase functional capacity in response to injury. Thus, a significant reduction in functioning renal mass (50-60%) may occur prior to the onset of any significant symptoms or even before any major biochemical alterations appear. Individual nephrons are able to adapt to nephron loss by increasing single nephron GFR (i.e. adaptive hyperfiltration). Although initially beneficial, hyperfiltration appears to result in long-term damage to the glomeruli of the remaining nephrons. In addition to the detrimental effects of acquired nephron loss, severe inborn deficits in total nephron load can also cause progressive glomerular injury. Nephrons may be lost via toxic, anoxic, or immunological injury, which may initially injure the glomerulus, the tubule, or both together. Glomerular damage can involve endothelial, epithelial, or mesangial cells, and/or the basement membrane. Inflammatory stimuli are released, including both cytokines and growth factors such as transforming growth factor beta (TGF-β), interleukin-6, interferon-γ, or tissue necrosis factor-α (TNF-α); these inflammatory factors activate resident lymphocytes and macrophages and recruit additional cells from the peripheral circulation. Thus, cellular infiltration is a common but not universal finding in kidney biopsy specimens. The activated cells can cause T-cell mediated cell lysis and activation and proliferation of interstitial fibroblasts. Fibroblast activity results in increased extracellular matrix synthesis and eventually glomerular and tubular fibrosis. The extracellular matrix expansion causes disruption of local blood flow, exaggerating regional ischemia, and a vicious cycle of inflammation, fibrosis and cell death is propagated.

Modifying progression
The most readily identifiable risk factors for progressive CKD (a decrease in GFR of greater than 5 mL/min/year corrected for body surface area) are hypertension and proteinuria. Typical goals for blood pressure are in the order of < 130 mmHg systolic blood pressure and < 80 mmHg diastolic pressure and even lower in proteinuric disease and diabetes-related kidney disease. The Modification of Diet in Renal Disease (MDRD) Study compared the rates of decline in GFR in 840 patients with various different causes of CKD to either a 'usual' or 'low' blood pressure goal. Patients with type 1 diabetes were excluded. Outcome data suggest that the low blood pressure goal had some beneficial effect in those patients with higher levels of proteinuria. The study supported the concept that proteinuria is an independent risk factor for progression of kidney disease. For patients with proteinuria of more than 1 g/24 h (approximately equivalent to 100 mg/mmol creatinine) the suggested target for mean blood pressure was 92 mmHg (125/75 mmHg). This target for blood pressure is lower than the recently published seventh report of the Joint National Committee on Prevention, Detection, Evaluation, and Treatment of High Blood Pressure (JNC-VII). In 2002, the UK Renal Association revised the target blood pressure to < 130/80 mmHg for stable CKD and < 125/75 mmHg for progressive CKD. Data from NHANES III revealed that among hypertensive individuals with an increased serum creatinine concentration, 75% were on antihypertensive treatment and only 11% had their blood pressure reduced to < 130/85 mm Hg.

ACE inhibitors are more effective than other antihypertensive drugs in slowing the rate of progression of proteinuric CKD. ACE inhibitors initially cause a mild decrease in GFR (< 10 mL/min/1.73 m^2). The development of hypotension, ARF, or severe hyperkalaemia (serum potassium concentration greater than 5.5 mmol/L) should prompt discontinuation of the drug until other causes have been excluded. Short-term studies show that ARBs have effects on blood pressure and proteinuria that are similar to those of ACE inhibitors. In addition, data from Japan have suggested that combining the two classes of drugs can give additional benefit than either drug alone in terms of reduction in proteinuria and progression to primary end-points.

The stage of kidney disease at presentation has an important bearing on the outcome of CKD. Patients with stage 4 and 5 CKD have a poor prognosis compared to those patients identified at earlier stages. This is not surprising since epidemiological data support the hypothesis that the vast majority of patients with stage 3 CKD do not develop progressive kidney failure and are more likely to die of comorbid diseases, particularly cardiovascular disease, than progress to stage 5 CKD. Factors associated with progression of CKD are summarised in Figure 2.7.

Risk factors for progression of kidney disease	
Non-modifiable	**Modifiable**
Reduction in nephron number (congenital or acquired)	Persistent activity of underlying disease
Increasing age	Inadequate control of hypertension
Ethnic group	Proteinuria > 1 g/24 h despite RAAS blockade
Chronic tubulointerstitial fibrosis at diagnosis (renal scarring)	Failure of adequate follow-up
	High protein diet
	Exposure to potentially nephrotoxic drugs
	Obesity
RAAS = renin-angiotensin-aldosterone system	

Figure 2.7 Risk factors for progression of kidney disease.

Further reading

Brenner BM. Retarding the progression of renal disease. Kidney Int 2003; **64:** 370-378.

Feehally J. Ethnicity and renal disease. Kidney Int 2005; **68:** 414-424.

Klahr S, Levey AS, Beck GJ, Caggiula AW, Hunsicker L, Kusek JW, *et al*. The effects of dietary protein restriction and blood-pressure control on the progression of chronic renal disease. Modification of Diet in Renal Disease Study Group. N Engl J Med 1994; **330:** 877-884.

Levey A, Eckardt K-U, Tsukamoto Y, Levin A *et al*. Definition and classification of chronic kidney disease: A position statement from Kidney Disease: Improving Global Outcomes (KDIGO). Kidney Int 2005; **67:** 2089-2100.

Chapter 3

Assessment of kidney function

Urinary examination

Urinalysis is invaluable in the identification of urological and kidney disease. Examination of a midstream urine sample is often the first step in the assessment of a patient suspected of having, or confirmed to have, deterioration in kidney function. The appearance of urine itself can be helpful, a darkening from the normal pale straw colour indicating a more concentrated urine or the presence of another pigment. A variety of foods and drugs may alter the colour of urine; for example beetroot and levodopa may impart red and brown coloration respectively. Haemoglobin and myoglobin can give a pink-red-brown coloration, depending on the concentration. Turbidity in a fresh sample may indicate urinary tract infection (UTI), but may also be due to fat particles in a patient with nephrotic syndrome. Excessive foaming of urine when shaken suggests proteinuria. Urine is often evaluated with the help of reagent strip ('dipstick') tests or examined microscopically.

Reagent strip ('dipstick') testing

Many tests of renal significance have been adapted for use on pads of cellulose (fixed on strips of plastic) that have been coated or impregnated with reagents for the analyte in question. Such dipstick tests may contain reagents for just one test per stick or for multiple tests on a single stick. Dipstick tests detect substances that overflow into the urine, such as glucose, ketones and urobilinogen, in addition to changes in constituents that are more directly linked to pathology affecting the kidneys or urinary tract. Urine samples for dipstick testing should be collected in sterile containers and dipstick testing performed on the fresh urine. Dipsticks should only be used if they have been stored correctly (i.e. desiccated), as they can deteriorate in a matter of hours. Testing urine for the presence of total protein, albumin and haemoglobin is considered elsewhere in this chapter. Comments on the principle and performance of other dipstick tests pertinent to the assessment of kidney function are given below. Dipstick urinalyses generally have poor sensitivity and specificity (Figure 3.1).

Leucocytes

Leucocyte esterase is produced by neutrophils and may signal pyuria associated with UTI. Pyuria is the presence of white blood cells in the urine. Significant pyuria is normally defined as a urinary white cell count ≥ 10 leucocytes/μL. The dipstick test for leucocytes uses an absorbent cellulose pad impregnated with a buffered mixture of derivatised pyrrole amino acid ester and diazonium salt. Leucocyte esterases catalyse the hydrolysis of the derivatised pyrrole amino acid ester to liberate 3-hydroxy-5-phenylpyrrole. This pyrrole then reacts with a diazonium salt to produce a purple product, the colour of which is compared with the colour chart. The test is claimed to have a detection limit of 5 to 15 cells/μL in urine and the darkest colour block is equivalent to 500 cells/μL or greater.

Causes of false-negative and false-positive urinalysis results

	False-positive for kidney disease	False-negative for kidney disease
Blood	Hypochlorite solutions Oxidising agents Bacterial peroxidase Menstrual contamination	Vitamin C Gentisic acid Poorly mixed urine
Leucocyte esterase	Contamination	High glucose concentration High specific gravity Cefalexin Tetracyclin Oxalic acid
Nitrites	Exposure of dipstick to air	High specific gravity Vitamin C
Protein	Infected (alkalinised) urine	Dilute urine Tubular proteinuria
Specific gravity[a]	Dextran solutions Radio-opaque dyes	Alkaline urine
General problems (may affect any of above)	Poor adherence to protocol (e.g. timing of reading) Colour blindness Sample or reagent strip storage issues	

[a]either falsely elevated (false-positive) or falsely depressed (false-negative)

Figure 3.1 Causes of false-negative and false-positive urinalysis results.
Only tests pertinent to the investigation of kidney disease are considered.

Nitrite

Nitrites are not normally present in urine but are found when bacteria reduce urinary nitrates to nitrites. Many Gram-negative and some Gram-positive organisms are capable of this conversion. To measure nitrite, the reagent pad is impregnated with p-arsanilic acid and tetrahydro-benzo(h)quinolin-3-ol. The reaction is based on arsanilic acid, in the presence of nitrite, converting to a diazonium salt, which couples with the quinolol to produce a pink colour. The detection limit of the test is 13 to 22 μmol/L nitrite in urine with a normal specific gravity. It will only measure nitrite and is claimed to detect populations of bacteria at a level of 10^5 colony forming units (CFU)/mL or more (N.B., by convention, UTI is commonly considered present when microbiological examination shows a pure growth of $\geq 10^5$ CFU/mL). The test may be less helpful in young children, in whom the urine remains in the bladder for less time, thereby limiting the time for nitrite production. The combination of the nitrite and leucocyte esterase tests is valuable in identifying patients with UTI, but negative results do not exclude UTI.

Specific gravity

Urinary specific gravity correlates with osmolality and gives an indication of urinary concentration. The test device for specific gravity consists of an absorbent cellulose pad impregnated with bromthymol blue, polymethylvinyl ether/maleic anhydride and sodium hydroxide. The test depends on the apparent pK_a change of the pretreated polyelectrolyte in relation to ionic strength; the hydrogen ions released are detected by the pH indicator. The colour changes from a dark blue at a low specific gravity (1.000) to yellow-green at a specific gravity of 1.030. Normal urinary specific gravity ranges from 1.003 to 1.030; higher values may indicate dehydration, glycosuria or the syndrome of inappropriate antidiuretic hormone. Low values are associated with conditions in which a concentrated urine cannot be formed (e.g. diuretic use, diabetes insipidus, adrenal insufficiency). In patients with intrinsic renal insufficiency the specific gravity becomes fixed at 1.010, reflecting the specific gravity of the glomerular filtrate.

pH

To measure the pH of a sample, the test pad is impregnated with indicators, one example being a mixture of methyl red and bromthymol blue. Methyl red in a diluted form is red at pH values below 4.2 and yellow at values above 6.2. Bromthymol blue is yellow at pH values below 6.0 and blue at values above 7.6. At pHs within these values, the indicators give shades of orange and green, respectively. It is important to recognise that the pH of urine alters with standing and the colour of the reagent blocks with time also; therefore, careful adherence to the recommended procedure is important. Urinary pH can range from 4.5 to 8.0, but is normally slightly acidic (5.5 to 6.5). Ingestion of proteins and acidic fruits (e.g. cranberry juice) can lower urinary pH whereas diets high in citrate tend to alkalinise urine. The measurement of urine pH can be helpful in the assessment of patients with renal tubular acidosis and in stone formers, although evaluation using a pH electrode may be more informative.

Microscopic examination of urine

Prior to examination, urine is centrifuged, the supernatant decanted and the sediment resuspended in the remaining liquid. A single drop of this suspension is transferred to a microscope slide for examination. Microscopic examination of a fresh urine sample will show the presence of a few cells (erythrocytes, leucocytes, and cells derived from the kidney and urinary tract), casts and, possibly, fat or pigmented particles. Casts are a coagulum of THG and the trapped contents of the tubular lumen. They originate from the distal convoluted tubule and the collecting duct during periods of urinary concentration or stasis and their cylindrical shape reflects that of the tubule in which they were formed. Inflammation of the upper urinary tract is associated with the presence of polymorphonuclear leucocytes and casts, whereas in lower urinary tract inflammation casts are absent. The presence of dysmorphic red cells may imply glomerular disease. In acute glomerulonephritis, haematuria may lead to coloration of the urine and the presence of large numbers of red and white blood cells; as the duration of the disease increases, the amount of sediment diminishes. The presence of bacteriuria is suggestive of UTI in males but clean-catch specimens from female patients are commonly contaminated by vaginal flora. Nephrologists will often describe urine as having either an 'active urinary sediment' or as 'bland'. An active urinary sediment means that signs of active kidney inflammation (red blood cells, white blood cells, casts) can be detected when the urine is examined under the microscope.

Proteinuria

Proteinuria is a common finding and an important prognostic indicator in patients with kidney disease. The use of a dipstick assay, with follow-up laboratory testing when indicated, has traditionally been used as a screening test in any patient suspected of having renal disease.

Physiology and pathology: types of proteinuria

Higher molecular weight proteins are largely retained within the circulation by the glomerular filter. Lower molecular weight proteins are more freely filtered, reabsorbed by proximal tubular cells and then catabolised within the tubular cells. The tubular reabsorptive process is saturable. The physiology of this process is described in Chapter 1.

Protein excretion displays considerable biological variability, and may be increased by upright posture, exercise, fever, UTI and heart failure as well as by kidney disease. Any increase in the filtered load (due to glomerular damage, increased glomerular vascular permeability or increased circulating concentration of low molecular weight proteins) or decrease in reabsorptive capacity (due to tubular damage) can result in increased urinary protein excretion (proteinuria). Consequently, the appearance of significant amounts of protein in the urine suggests kidney disease. Proteinuria is commonly classified as either tubular or glomerular depending on the pattern of proteinuria observed. A third category, overflow proteinuria, is also recognised, in which filtration of excessive amounts of low molecular weight protein exceeds the tubular capacity for reabsorption (Figure 3.2).

Characterisation of proteinuria

Type of proteinuria	Causes	Examples of proteins seen
Glomerular	Increased glomerular permeability	Progressively increasing excretion of higher molecular weight proteins as permeability increases (e.g. albumin, IgG)
Tubular	Proximal tubular damage: decreased tubular reabsorptive capacity and/or release of intra-cellular components (e.g. due to nephrotoxic drugs)	α_1-microglobulin β_2-microglobulin Retinol binding protein Enzymuria (e.g. *N*-acetyl-β-D-glucosaminidase, alkaline phosphatase) α-glutathione-S-transferase
	Decreased nephron number: increased filtered load per nephron	As above
	Distal tubular damage	Tamm-Horsfall glycoprotein π-glutathione-S-transferase
Overflow	Increased plasma concentration of relatively freely filtered protein	Bence Jones protein Lysozyme Myoglobin

Figure 3.2 Characterisation of proteinuria

GLOMERULAR PROTEINURIA

Any glomerular disease process may increase glomerular permeability either as a consequence of podocyte foot process retraction and effacement or basement membrane damage from, for example, deposition of immune complexes or increased matrix protein deposition, as in diabetic nephropathy, or both (see Chapter 5). Altered glomerular permeability increases the filtered load of all proteins, but the most characteristic feature is the increasing amount of the higher molecular weight proteins, such as albumin, in the urine. As permeability increases, progressively larger proteins (e.g. IgG) will be excreted in larger amounts (non-selective proteinuria).

TUBULAR PROTEINURIA

This is seen in the presence of decreased tubular reabsorptive capacity and/or tubular damage with essentially normal glomerular permeability. Proximal tubular cells may be damaged by toxic agents (e.g. drugs, heavy metals) or by anoxia, resulting in decreased reabsorption of filtered proteins. Lower molecular weight proteins (e.g. RBP, α_1-microglobulin) appear in relatively higher amounts in the urine than albumin, producing a so-called tubular proteinuria pattern. Albumin itself also normally undergoes extensive tubular reabsorption (see below). The reason why albumin excretion is not consistently increased in this setting is unclear, but it has been suggested that the endocytic uptake process is mediated by receptor(s) with differing affinities for different proteins (or classes of proteins), with albumin being preferentially reabsorbed.

Damage to tubular epithelial cells causes not only functional disturbances but also structural change, with increased cellular turnover and cell lysis resulting in the release of both brush border (e.g. alkaline phosphatase) and lysosomal enzymes (e.g. N-acetyl-β-D-glucosaminidase [NAG]). Measurement of α- and π-glutathione-S-transferase isoenzymes has been proposed to discriminate between proximal and distal tubular damage respectively, but the role of these markers in clinical practice has yet to be established. THG, derived from the thick ascending limb of the loop of Henle and the early distal convoluted tubule, has also been used as a marker of more distal tubular damage.

CKD is invariably accompanied by a decrease in the number of viable nephrons. There is a compensatory increase in glomerular filtration in the remaining glomeruli resulting in an increased filtered load of protein per nephron. In the absence of glomerular permeability changes, this will also give a tubular protein-uria pattern. Leakage of various plasma proteins into the urinary space as a result of tubulointerstitial damage may also occur. This can cause haematuria and proteinuria in the absence of changes in glomerular permeability or tubular reab-sorption.

OVERFLOW PROTEINURIA

The selective increase in the urinary excretion of an individual low molecular weight protein suggests that its production rate, and thus plasma concentration, has increased dramatically without concomitant glomerular or tubular damage. Examples of this are the urinary excretion of myoglobin, lysozyme and immunoglobulin light chains (Bence Jones protein, BJP). Myoglobin is a small (17.8 kDa), haem-containing protein normally catabolised by endocytosis and proteolysis in the proximal tubule following glomerular filtration. Typically only 0.01-5.0% of filtered protein appears in the urine. However, following rhabdomyolysis large amounts of myoglobin are released into the plasma, saturating the tubular reabsorptive mechanism and resulting in the appearance of significant quantities of myoglobin in the urine. Furthermore, myoglobin is directly toxic to the renal tubules and can cause acute tubular necrosis with ARF. A variety of approaches can be used to quantitate or detect myoglobin in the urine, but for most clinical purposes evidence that rhabdomyolysis has occurred is better demonstrated by an increase in serum creatine kinase activity not attributable to a cardiac source. Urinary myoglobin measurement provides no additional prognostic or diagnostic information in this setting. Lysozyme is an enzyme that occurs in neutrophilic granulocytes, monocytes, and macrophages, as well as several organs of the body, including the spleen, kidney, and gastrointestinal tract. It is freely filtered by the kidney and absorbed by the proximal tubules. Thus, lysozymuria is seen in conditions associated with both tubular damage and increased endogenous synthesis; its primary clinical application has been in the monitoring of patients with monocytic leukaemia. The clinical significance of urinary BJP (22 kDa) is discussed in Chapter 5.

Sample collection

There has been extensive discussion in the literature about the appropriate urine sample to use for the investigation of protein excretion. Commonly, a 24 h urine sample is used as the definitive means of demonstrating the presence of proteinuria, although this is an imperfect reference method. It is widely accepted that this is a difficult procedure to control effectively; studies have shown that more than 25% of samples have to be discarded because an incomplete collection is suspected. Overnight, first void in the morning ('early morning urine', EMU), second void in the morning, or random sample collections have also been used. Since creatinine excretion in the urine is fairly constant throughout the 24 h period, measurement of protein:creatinine ratios allows correction for variations in urinary concentration. Furthermore, the protein:creatinine ratio has been shown to give at least equivalent power to 24 h urinary protein excretion as a predictor of the rate of loss of GFR in non-diabetic nephropathy. In practice, for screening purposes, spot urine protein:creatinine ratios can be used to rule out the need for 24 h collections, which are generally not necessary; this practice has been endorsed by the NSF for Renal

Disease. An early morning urine sample is preferred since it correlates well with 24 h protein excretion and is required to exclude the diagnosis of orthostatic (postural) proteinuria. However, a random urine sample is acceptable if no early morning sample is available. If required, daily protein excretion (in mg/24 h) can be roughly estimated by multiplying the protein:creatinine ratio (measured in mg/mmol) by a factor of 10 since, although daily excretion of creatinine depends on muscle mass, an average figure of 10 mmol creatinine/24 h can be assumed. Clearly, the use of this number will lead to overestimation of daily protein excretion in patients with low muscle mass and underestimation in patients with high muscle mass; in addition, there may be racial variation in creatinine excretion even after adjustment for muscle mass. Figure 3.3 explains the relationship between urinary protein (and albumin) concentrations expressed as a ratio to creatinine and other common expressions of their concentration. A suitable protocol for the further investigation of patients found to have proteinuria at screening is given in Figure 3.4.

Urinary protein concentration and clinical correlates

	Urine reagent strip ('dipstick') reading[a]	Urine protein: creatinine ratio mg/mmol (urine protein mg/L)	Urine total protein excretion mg/24 h (g/24 h)	Urinary albumin: creatinine ratio mg/mmol	Urinary albumin excretion µg/min (mg/24 h)
Normal	Negative	<15 (<100)	<150 (<0.15)	≤2.5 (males) ≤3.5 (females)	≤20 (≤30)
Microalbuminuria 'Trace' protein	Negative Trace	<15 (<100) 15-49 (100-329)	<150 (<0.15) 150-499 (0.15-0.499)	2.6 - 29 (males) 3.6 - 29 (females)	21-199 (31-299)
Clinical proteinuria (macroalbuminuria)	+	50-149 (330-999)	500-1499 (0.500-1.499)	≥30	≥200 (≥300)
	++	150-449 (1000-2999)	1500-4499 (1.500-4.499)		
Nephrotic range	+++	≥450 (≥3000)	≥4500 (≥4.5)		

[a]These are typical values; some reagent strip manufacturers may use different values

Figure 3.3 Expressions of urinary protein concentration and their approximate equivalents and clinical correlates. The table assumes an average creatinine excretion of 10 mmol/24 h and an average urine volume of 1.5 L/24 h. Males and females have different thresholds for the diagnosis of microalbuminuria as a consequence of the lower urinary creatinine excretion in women.

Investigation of a patient with positive dipstick for urine protein

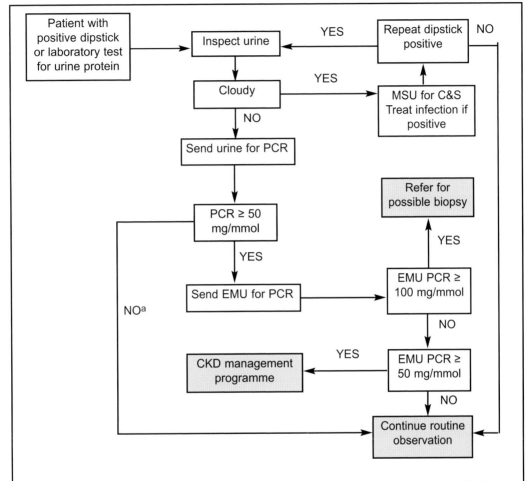

a In the absence of a systemic disease such as diabetes or hypertension, a borderline elevation in total protein excretion (15-49 mg/mmol), without haematuria or a rise in serum creatinine concentration, is unlikely to be associated with a serious primary renal pathology.

Figure 3.4 Suggested protocol for the further investigation of patients found to have a positive (+ or above) dipstick or quantitative protein test.

Reagent strip ('dipstick') testing devices show both false negatives and false positives: positive results should therefore be confirmed using laboratory testing on at least two further occasions. Patients with two or more positive (> 50 mg total protein/mmol creatinine) quantitative tests spaced by 1-2 weeks should be diagnosed as having persistent proteinuria. Postural proteinuria should be excluded by the examination of an early morning urine (EMU).

C&S, culture and sensitivity; CKD, chronic kidney disease; MSU, mid-stream urine; PCR, protein:creatinine ratio

Measurement of total protein

Urinary total protein concentration can be estimated using reagent strip ('dipstick') test devices or measured by a variety of laboratory techniques. Dipstick testing for proteinuria is inadequate in patients with diabetes, who should undergo annual testing for microalbuminuria (see below). Because standard urine dipsticks rely on estimation of protein concentration, which in turn depends on hydration (i.e. how concentrated the urine sample is), these tests can only give a rough indication of the presence or absence of pathological proteinuria.

The dipstick test for total protein includes a cellulose test pad impregnated with tetrabromphenol blue and a citrate pH 3 buffer. The reaction is based on the 'protein error of indicators' phenomenon in which certain chemical indicators demonstrate one colour in the presence of protein and another in its absence. Thus, tetrabromphenol blue is green in the presence of protein at pH 3 but yellow in its absence. The colour is read after exactly 60 s and the test has a lower detection limit of 150 to 300 mg/L, depending on the types and proportions of protein present. The reagent is most sensitive to albumin and less sensitive to globulins, Bence Jones protein, THG, and haemoglobin. Typically, a colour matching the 'trace' block on the dipstick corresponds to approximately 150 mg/L of total protein and a colour matching the '+' block to 300 mg/L. Significant ('clinical') proteinuria is deemed to be present when the colour change matches any block greater than that of the trace block (i.e. > 300 mg/L); assuming a typical urinary volume of 1.5 L/24 h, this is approximately equivalent to a total protein excretion of 500 mg/24 h (~ 50 mg/mmol creatinine). However, the specificity of urinalysis using protein dipsticks for the detection of proteinuria is poor and misclassification errors are common (Figure 3.1). Positive dipstick tests should be confirmed in the laboratory by measuring either the protein:creatinine or albumin:creatinine ratio on an early morning or random urine sample. A creatinine test pad (using the peroxidase-like activity of transition metal creatinine complexes) has been added to some strip systems to enable a ratio of protein (or albumin) to creatinine to be reported in order to reduce the intra-individual variation seen with random urine collections.

Laboratory methods used for the measurement of urinary total protein include the original Lowry method, turbidimetry after mixing with trichloroacetic or sulphosalicylic acid, turbidimetry with benzethonium chloride (benzyl-dimethyl {2-[2-(p-1,1,3,3-tetramethyl-butylphenoxy)ethoxy]ethyl}ammonium chloride) and dye binding with Coomassie Brilliant Blue or pyrogallol red molybdate. Concerns about variation in the response to different proteins have led to many variants of the methods being published. The turbidimetric methods and the dye-binding methods do not give equal analytical specificity and sensitivity for all proteins;

this may be of particular importance in the detection of light chains, when an immunochemical method is more appropriate. External quality assessment programmes have highlighted significant variation between methods and, in particular, poor precision at low concentrations.

Measurement of specific proteins

Chromatographic and electrophoretic (including capillary electrophoresis) techniques can provide a semi-quantitative or qualitative measurement of the range of proteins appearing in the urine and estimations of a panel or pattern of proteins that are not as easily available with individual assays. Immunoassay is the preferred method for the accurate, precise and sensitive quantitation of individual proteins. A variety of analytical approaches can be used but the most common approach today employs a light-scattering immunoassay, with either turbidimetric or nephelometric detection of immunoaggregate formation. In addition to albumin, immunoassay techniques are used to measure low molecular weight proteins in urine, most commonly α_1-microglobulin and RBP. In the past there has been considerable study of the excretion of β_2-microglobulin; however, it is an impractical marker because of its instability in urine at a pH of less than 6. α_1-microglobulin (31 kDa) is also referred to as protein HC because of its human complex-forming capacity with IgA. It is synthesised by the liver and the free form is readily filtered at the glomerulus. RBP (22 kDa) is also synthesised by the liver and is found in the plasma as a complex with prealbumin; the protein is the carrier protein for vitamin A. For the identification of tubular damage, urinary RBP may be more sensitive than α_1-microglobulin, but the higher concentration and excellent stability of the latter in human urine *ex vivo* facilitates its use as a marker of tubular damage in clinical studies.

The enzyme NAG is stable in urine and has been used as a marker of tubular integrity in a variety of diseases associated with renal injury, including hypertension, drug nephrotoxicity, transplantation, and diabetic nephropathy. One method for the assay of NAG employs the substrate 4-methylumbelliferyl-N-acetyl-β-D-glucosaminide with fluorometric detection of the methylumbelliferone released by the enzyme. Alternative substrates generating products capable of being detected in the visible spectrum have also been described. However, while it is a sensitive marker of kidney damage, it has not generally been shown to provide any clear benefit over other markers of tubular proteinuria.

Although a variety of tests have been used for the detection of BJP, including the classic heat test and the Bradshaw test, electrophoresis supplemented by immunofixation is the most reliable approach. Quantitation of BJP excretion may be required when monitoring patients with light chain only myeloma; although imperfect, this is currently best achieved by electrophoresis and densitometry although recently described immunoassays for free light chains in serum and urine may also have a role in this setting.

Indications for urinary protein measurement

Proteinuria is a potent risk marker for both progressive kidney disease (diabetic and non-diabetic) and cardiovascular disease; reduction of protein excretion is a therapeutic target. Investigation for increased urinary protein excretion is mandatory in any patient with suspected kidney disease. In the international classification of CKD, stage 1 and 2 CKD require the presence of a marker of kidney damage other than altered GFR; proteinuria is the most important and frequent of these markers. Among patients with suspected or proven CKD, including reflux nephropathy, early glomerulonephritis and those with hypertension, annual urinalysis for proteinuria is accepted as a useful way of identifying patients at risk of progressive kidney disease. The presence of proteinuria is highly predictive of significant glomerular disease amongst patients with haematuria. Although patients with macroscopic haematuria will be referred first for urological evaluation, the presence of proteinuria accompanying macroscopic haematuria greatly increases the probability that the patient will turn out to have glomerular disease, most commonly IgA nephropathy/glomerulonephritis. Urinalysis is widely used both in primary care and in hospital practice and can be very useful in the initial investigation of systemic illness, where a positive protein result should lead to active consideration of rapidly progressive glomerulonephritis. Haematuria and proteinuria are almost universally found in acute glomerulonephritis, whether primary or secondary to systemic disease (e.g. vasculitis, SLE, cryoglobulinaemia). Proteinuria is the hallmark of renal amyloidosis. Some neoplastic processes cause paraneoplastic kidney disease, which is also classically associated with proteinuria.

Proteinuria is therefore important both for the identification of kidney damage and for guiding future treatment and surveillance. Urinary protein measurement should be undertaken in the following situations:

- newly discovered increased serum creatinine concentration/reduced GFR
- assessment of severity of known kidney disease
- newly discovered haematuria
- initial assessment of patients with hypertension
- in patients with unexplained oedema
- in patients with cardiovascular disease
- suspected multisystem disease (e.g. SLE)
- family history of stage 5 CKD or hereditary kidney disease
- structural renal tract disease, recurrent renal calculi or prostatic hypertrophy

Significance of proteinuria: equivalence with albuminuria

Proteinuria ≥ 500 mg/24 h is generally pathological, especially if there is concomitant haematuria. However, there are exceptions to this. Proteinuria can occur as a result of fever and exercise (functional) or be related to posture (orthostatic). These sporadic changes can cause interpretative difficulties when pathology is suspected. Upright posture increases protein excretion in both normal subjects and those with kidney disease. If proteinuria is postural, disappearing during recumbency and absent from early morning samples, the patient can be strongly reassured. In these benign situations the level of proteinuria rarely exceeds 1000 mg/24 h (~100 mg/mmol creatinine). Proteinuria above 1000 mg/24 h implies glomerular proteinuria. Glomerular proteinuria may be heavy and a mixed proteinuria with elevation of both high and low molecular weight proteins may be observed. Numerous studies have demonstrated that proteinuria is a potent risk marker for progression of renal disease; at all levels of GFR, the concomitant presence of proteinuria greatly increases the risk of progressive disease.

As discussed above, both laboratory measurements of urinary total protein and conventional urine dipsticks show differential reactivity with albumin and other proteins present in urine. The relationship between albumin and total protein excretion changes in disease, with increasing proteinuria largely reflecting albuminuria; typically albumin represents approximately 20% of total urinary protein at 150 mg/L, 50% at 300 mg/L and 70% at 1000 mg/L. This causes difficulties when trying to reconcile the literature pertaining to pathological proteinuria and albuminuria, in particular when comparing studies on diabetic and non-diabetic nephropathy. Whilst the diagnosis of clinical proteinuria in the non-diabetic population has traditionally been based on 'dipstick positivity', in the diabetic population definitions of proteinuria (sometimes termed 'macroalbuminuria') have tended to evolve based upon urinary albumin excretion as a result of the staging system for diabetic nephropathy (see Chapter 5). There is no definitive level of albuminuria equivalent to the cut-off point for proteinuria in the literature. Hence, definitions of proteinuria are not always consistent between the diabetic and non-diabetic populations. In the UK, the National Institute for Health and Clinical Excellence (NICE) has defined proteinuria in diabetes as an albumin concentration in excess of 200 mg/L or > 30 mg/mmol creatinine or an excretion rate of > 300 mg/24 h (approximating 200 μg/min). The equivalences of these thresholds generally assume an average urinary volume of 1.5 L/24 h and an average creatinine excretion of 10 mmol/24 h. These definitions are broadly in keeping with North American definitions of macroalbuminuria. In the non-diabetic population, proteinuria is typically considered to be present when total protein exceeds 500 mg/24 h or 50 mg/mmol. Cut-offs of ≥ 50 mg/mmol and ≥ 30 mg/mmol for total protein or albumin respectively are only approximately equivalent (Figure 3.3). In practice, in non-diabetic patients in the absence of concomitant haematuria, proteinuria does not generally act as a trigger for active intervention until the ratio exceeds 100 mg/mmol (approximately ++ on dipstick testing).

Several groups have demonstrated that urinary total protein measurement can be replaced by that of albumin. This may provide a more specific and sensitive measure of changes in glomerular permeability, although it should also be noted that changes in albumin excretion may reflect overall changes in vascular permeability and therefore may not indicate an explicit deterioration in renal function. Furthermore, measurement of urine albumin concentration is more expensive than measurement of urine total protein and may be misleading in tubular disease. Many of the previous studies of the natural history or treatment of kidney disease stratified patients by total protein excretion, rather than by albumin excretion. NICE has recommended that to detect proteinuria the urinary albumin:creatinine ratio should be used in preference to other tests of proteinuria, including the protein:creatinine ratio and reagent strip testing (see Chapter 8). It is increasingly accepted that proteinuria is not just a consequence of, but contributes directly to, progression of kidney disease. The accumulation of proteins in abnormal amounts in the tubular lumen may trigger an inflammatory reaction that contributes to interstitial structural damage and expansion, and progression of kidney disease. Evidence gathered from *in vitro* studies suggests that glomerular filtration of an abnormal amount or types of protein induces mesangial cell injury, leading to glomerulosclerosis, and that these same proteins can also have adverse effects on proximal tubular cell function. The use of ACE inhibitors and ARBs, either alone or in combination, reduces protein excretion by reducing intraglomerular filtration pressure and, possibly, by stabilising the glomerular epithelial cell slit diaphragm proteins. Consequently, reduction of proteinuria is an important therapeutic target.

Albuminuria

Physiology and pathology: definition of microalbuminuria

Human albumin has a molecular mass of 66 kDa and is negatively charged at physiological pH. It is extensively retained by the glomerulus, with its filtration fraction (0.004) being much lower than that of a neutral dextran of the same radius; the negative charge of albumin confers on it the filtration properties of a larger molecule, resulting in virtual exclusion of albumin from the urinary space. Nevertheless, approximately 1.3 g/24 h of albumin passes through the glomerular capillary walls. The majority of this is taken up by endosomes in the proximal tubular cells. The endosomes merge with lysosomes where albumin is digested, particularly by cysteine proteases, into 0.5 to 1.5 kDa fragments. Most of these fragments are released into the renal vein, conserving amino acids in the body. In health, small quantities (approximately 15 mg/24 h) of intact albumin appear in the urine. Small amounts of the digested albumin fragments may also be released into the tubular lumen and appear in the urine. 'Microalbuminuria' is a term for the excretion of albumin in the urine in amounts that are abnormal, but below the limit of detection of conventional urine dipsticks and only therefore detected by specific tests for albumin. The term is confusing in that it can mistakenly be taken to mean that there is abnormal excretion of 'microalbumin', (i.e. a small albumin molecule), whereas in fact the albumin excreted in this condition is exactly the same as in other conditions that cause proteinuria. In 'overt diabetic nephropathy' the amount of albumin present in the urine reaches concentrations that can be detected by conventional urine dipsticks (Figure 3.3).

Sample collection
Urinary albumin should be measured in an early morning (preferred) or random mid-stream urine sample and is commonly expressed as an albumin:creatinine ratio. The diagnosis of microalbuminuria requires the demonstration of increased albumin excretion (either increased albumin:creatinine ratio or increased albumin excretion rate) in at least two out of three urine samples collected in the absence of infection or an acute metabolic crisis. Establishing the diagnosis has both prognostic and management implications in the care of patients with diabetes mellitus. The best possible metabolic control of diabetes should be achieved before investigating patients for micro-albuminuria. Patients should not be screened during intercurrent illness.

Measurement
Albumin is readily measured by quantitative immunoassay methods capable of detecting urinary albumin at low concentrations. Point of care testing devices have also been described for urinary albumin; some of these measure both albumin and creatinine, enabling calculation of the albumin:creatinine ratio.

Indications
Patients with diabetes mellitus who have persistent proteinuria do not require testing for microalbuminuria. All other patients with diabetes mellitus should undergo, as a minimum, annual testing for microalbuminuria. Screening should commence five years after diagnosis in patients with type 1 diabetes mellitus and at diagnosis in patients with type 2 diabetes without proteinuria and should continue on an annual basis up to the age of 75 years. A suitable protocol for microalbuminuria screening is shown in Figure 3.5. There is currently no proven role for screening for microalbuminuria in patients who do not have diabetes. Although microalbuminuria may act as a cardiovascular risk marker in non-diabetic people, particularly among hypertensive patients, and may also be a marker of early non-diabetic kidney disease, there is as yet no evidence that iden-

tification of such people would have implications for treatment over and above treatment of modifiable cardiovascular risk factors such as hyperlipidaemia, smoking, and hypertension.

Screening for microalbuminuria in diabetes mellitus

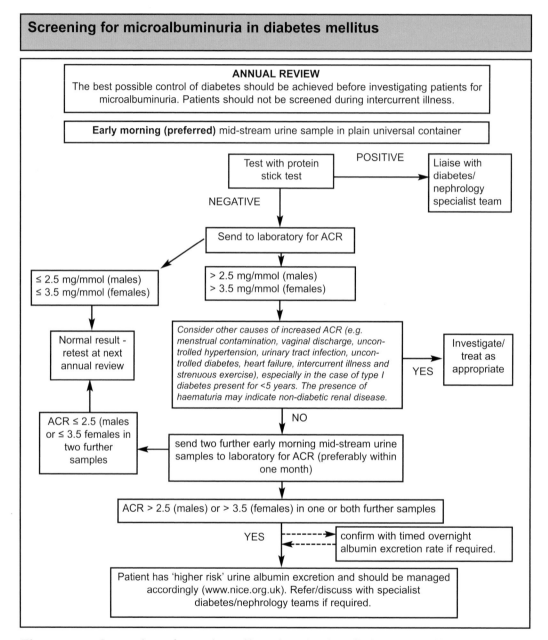

Figure 3.5 Screening for microalbuminuria in diabetes mellitus. Patients demonstrating 'higher risk' urinary albumin excretion should be managed accordingly (see Type 2 diabetes, Clinical Guidelines 66 @ www.nice.org.uk).

Significance of albuminuria

An albumin:creatinine ratio ≤ 2.5 mg/mmol in a male or ≤ 3.5 mg/mmol in a female requires no further investigation until the patient's next annual review. Patients demonstrating albumin:creatinine ratios above this cut-off should have urine samples sent to the laboratory on two further occasions (ideally within one month) for albumin estimation. Patients demonstrating increased albumin:creatinine ratios in one or both of these further samples have microalbuminuria. It is important to consider other causes of increased albumin excretion, especially in the case of type 1 diabetes present for < 5 years. These can include non-diabetic renal disease, menstrual contamination, vaginal discharge, uncontrolled hypertension, UTI, uncontrolled diabetes, heart failure, intercurrent illness and strenuous exercise. Occasionally, it may be desirable to confirm the diagnosis by measuring albumin excretion rate in a timed overnight collection: increased albumin excretion in an overnight collection is defined as an overnight albumin excretion rate > 20 µg/min (Figure 3.3).

The recognition of microalbuminuria in patients with diabetes mellitus allows identification of diabetic nephropathy, and institution of treatment to reduce the risk of progressive kidney damage and cardiovascular mortality, at an earlier stage than would be possible with conventional protein dipstick testing. Conventionally, in this clinical situation the aims of treatment differ according to the presence or absence of microalbuminuria or clinical proteinuria (see Chapter 5). However, it has also been argued that microalbuminuria may represent a false boundary in respect to institution of intensified therapy, there being no evidence that normoalbuminuric patients do not derive equivalent benefits from such treatments.

Haematuria

The presence of haemoglobin or red blood cells in the urine may be due to glomerular, tubulointerstitial, or postrenal (e.g. bladder) disease, although the latter two causes are the more common. Haematuria can be present in a range of kidney diseases, including glomerulonephritis (especially IgA nephropathy), polycystic kidney disease, sickle cell disease, vasculitis, and a range of infections. A spectrum of urological diseases may also give rise to haematuria, including bladder, prostate and pelvic/ureteric malignancy, kidney stones, trauma, bladder damage and ureteric stricture. Glomerular and tubulointerstitial haematuria are generally associated with proteinuria, although 20% of patients with glomerulonephritis present with haematuria alone. Postrenal haematuria is generally not associated with proteinuria.

Dipstick urinalysis is the test of choice for confirmation of macroscopic haematuria and for detection of microscopic haematuria. The presence of blood in the urine can be detected by the use of a phase contrast microscope to determine the presence of red cells in the urine sediment. However, this is seldom necessary in routine clinical practice. Although false positive dipstick tests for haematuria have been described, false negative microscopy in the routine microbiology laboratory is also common, due to lysis of red blood cells during transit, particularly in dilute urine. The diagnostic yield of investigation of patients with dipstick positive haematuria is similar whether or not haematuria is reported on microscopy. Infection, trauma, and menstruation should be excluded before confirmation of haematuria.

In the dipstick test for haemoglobin, the reagent pad is impregnated with buffered tetramethyl benzidine (TMB) and an organic peroxide. The method depends on detection of the peroxidase activity of haemoglobin, which catalyses the reaction of cumene hydroperoxide and TMB. The colour change ranges from orange through pale to dark green, and red cells or free haemoglobin are detected together with myoglobin. Two reagent pads are employed for the low haemoglobin level; if intact red cells are present, the low-level pad will have a speckled appearance, with a solid colour indicating haemolysed red cells. The detection limit for free haemoglobin is 150 to 600 μg/L or 5 to 20 intact red cells/μL. The test is equally sensitive to haemoglobin and myoglobin. Water must not be used as a negative control with this test due to the matrix requirements of the assay, as it will give a false positive result.

Testing for haematuria is indicated as part of the initial assessment of patients with:

- newly found increased serum creatinine concentration/reduced GFR
- newly discovered proteinuria
- suspected multisystem disease with possible renal involvement.

Patients with macroscopic haematuria should be referred to a urology service. The management of patients with microscopic haematuria is affected by whether they are also proteinuric. The prognosis for the combination of proteinuria with haematuria is significantly worse than that for proteinuria alone. Detection of haematuria in patients with abnormal GFR or proteinuria aids the identification of those with diseases such as glomerulonephritis (which may be secondary to systemic conditions such as vasculitis or SLE). The presence of haematuria in a patient with diabetes mellitus and microalbuminuria or proteinuria may be a marker of the presence of non-diabetic kidney disease and is considered by NICE as an indication for referral to a nephrology service. There is currently no evidence supporting screening of unselected populations for haematuria using dipstick testing.

Glomerular filtration rate

GFR as a measure of nephron function

Although the kidney has numerous functions, the initiating step in many of these processes is glomerular filtration. Each nephron produces about 100 μL of ultra-filtrate/24 h which, assuming an average of one million nephrons per kidney, on a whole body basis equates to approximately 200 L/24 h of ultrafiltrate, or 140 mL/min. The rate of ultrafiltration is known as the GFR and, in health, is therefore approximately 140 mL/min in the adult human. The GFR is widely accepted as the best overall measure of kidney function, enabling a statement of the complex functions of the kidney in a single numerical expression. A decrease in GFR precedes renal failure in all forms of progressive kidney disease, with different kidney pathologies progressing to end stage renal failure (ERF) and dialysis dependency at rates varying from weeks to several decades. The symptoms accompanying progressive kidney disease (including anaemia, hyperparathyroidism and cardiovascular disease) relate more closely to GFR than to serum creatinine concentration. Measuring GFR is useful in identifying CKD in order to (a) target treatment to prevent progression and complications and (b) to monitor progression and predict the point at which renal replacement therapy (RRT) will be required. It is also used as a guide for dosage of renally excreted drugs to avoid potential drug toxicity.

The GFR is a measure of the efficiency with which substances are cleared from the blood by glomerular filtration, and is defined as 'the volume of plasma from which a given substance is completely cleared by glomerular filtration per unit time'. It is measured by quantitating the clearance of an exogenous or endogenous substance by the kidneys. Provided that the substance (S) is in stable concentration in the plasma, is physiologically inert, freely filtered at the glomerulus, and neither secreted, reabsorbed, synthesised, nor metabolised by the kidney, then the amount of that substance filtered at the glomerulus is equal to the amount excreted in the urine (i.e. the amount of S entering the kidney must exactly equal the amount leaving it). The amount of S filtered at the glomerulus = GFR multiplied by plasma S concentration: $GFR \times [S]_p$. The amount of S excreted equals the urine S concentration ($[S]_u$) multiplied by the urinary flow rate (V, volume excreted per unit time). Since filtered S = excreted S:

$$GFR \times [S]_p = [S]_u \times V$$

which rearranges to:

$$GFR = ([S]_u \times V)/[S]_p$$

where GFR = *clearance* in units of mL of plasma cleared of a substance per minute
$[S]_u$ = urinary concentration of the substance
V = flow rate of urine in mL per min
$[S]_p$ = plasma concentration of the substance

The term $([S]_u \times V)/[S]_p$ is defined as the clearance of substance S and is an accurate estimate of GFR providing the aforementioned criteria are satisfied.

Within the animal kingdom, GFR is proportional to $(M)^{0.77}$, where M is body mass; metabolic rate is similarly related to body mass with an exponent of 0.75. In humans, GFR varies enormously with body size over a range from < 10 mL/min in neonates to 200 mL/min in large adults. To enable comparisons of GFR between individuals it has become standard practice to normalise GFR to a measure of body size. In healthy humans of different ages and body sizes, both the basal metabolic rate and the weight of the kidney are proportional to body surface area (BSA). It is therefore this measure that is generally used to adjust GFR when the aim is to express how close renal excretory function is to normal. In 1916 Delafield and Eugene Du Bois described a formula that enabled the estimation of BSA using power functions of height and weight:

$$BSA (m^2) = [weight (kg)^{0.425}] \times [height (cm)^{0.725}] \times 0.007184$$

Their formula was validated in nine subjects and has entered medical practice as the standard method by which BSA should be estimated in adults, although other formulae validated in larger populations have been described. Conventionally GFR is corrected to a BSA value of 1.73 m^2, representing the average BSA of adults aged 25 years:

$$GFR_{corrected} = GFR_{measured} \times (1.73/BSA\ m^2)$$

Measurement of GFR using exogenous substances
Measurement of GFR using an exogenous molecule enables small deteriorations in renal function to be observed even when the imprecision in measurement is taken into account. A variety of exogenous (non-radioisotopic and radioisotopic) markers have been used to estimate clearance. The use of exogenous markers to measure GFR is recommended for the monitoring of slowly progressing nephropathies such as that associated with diabetes mellitus and for evaluating renal function in potential kidney donors. Exogenous markers are also used to determine a GFR that is a benchmark against which to monitor deterioration in GFR using an endogenous marker such as creatinine.

GFR measurements can be based either on the urinary or plasma clearance of the marker. To ensure accuracy when measuring GFR using urinary clearance methods it is essential that (1) renal tubular secretion or reabsorption does not contribute to the elimination of the compound, (2) plasma protein binding of the pharmaceutical compound is negligible, and (3) patients completely empty their bladder. Plasma clearance of exogenous compounds measures GFR reliably only if non-renal clearance routes are negligible. For research purposes, in patients with low (< 30 mL/min) GFR and in patients with ascites or oedema, measurement is best performed using a urinary clearance method. From a clinical management perspective, either urinary or plasma clearance approaches are acceptable in the majority of patients.

Either constant infusion or single bolus injection methods may be used to administer exogenous markers. In the constant infusion technique, the fasting subject is required to drink 500 mL of water 1 h before the study begins after which he or she is required to take 200 mL every half hour until the end of the study. The subject remains supine throughout the study. An intravenous loading dose of the marker selected is then followed by a constant infusion of a given quantity of marker per minute for 3 h. After equilibration for 1 h, blood is taken and urine samples are collected at hourly intervals for 3 h. This technique can be used with any of the exogenous markers, the dosage being all that will vary between molecules. For example, for inulin an intravenous loading dose of 2.3 g would be followed by a constant infusion of 18.1 mg/min for 3 h.

Single bolus plasma clearance methods have obvious practical advantages compared to the complex continuous infusion methods. A single dose of the marker (e.g. inulin, 70 mg/kg; iohexol, 5 mL, [Omnipaque 300 mg iodine/mL, Nycomed AS, Oslo, Norway]; or ^{51}Cr-ethylenediaminetetraacetic acid [EDTA], 50-100 µCi) is injected and venous blood samples are then collected at timed intervals (e.g. typically 120, 180, and 240 min after the start of the injection for ^{51}Cr-EDTA). The GFR is calculated using knowledge of the amount of marker injected and the decrease in marker concentration (activity) as a function of time. The elimination of the marker is described by a two-compartment model; this comprises an initial equilibration or distribution phase while the marker mixes between the vascular and extravascular space while also being cleared from the plasma by the kidney. The distribution phase can last between 2 and 8 h, depending on the size of the subject, the distribution volume of the molecule (e.g. longer in oedematous patients), and the GFR of the subject (the lower the GFR, the longer the distribution phase). This gives rise to a bi-exponential clearance curve (Figure 3.6). However, GFR is normally calculated using single-exponential analysis by plotting log marker concentration against time. The half-life is calculated from the slope (k) and the volume of distribution (C_0) of the marker just after injection.

$$GFR = k \times C_0$$

Because this model ignores the distribution phase, GFR is overestimated. Various mathematical corrections can be used to adjust for this; those proposed by Chantler and Barrett and by Brochner-Mortensen have been widely used.

Plasma disappearance curve of a GFR marker

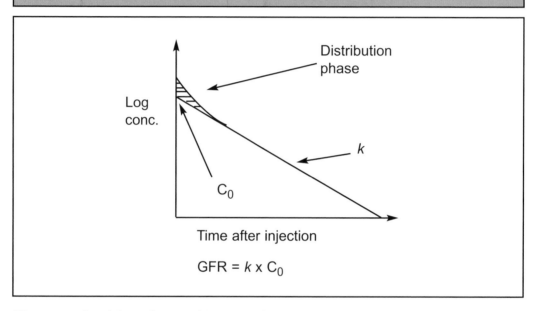

Figure 3.6 Semi-log plot used in a single compartmental analysis of the plasma disappearance curve of a glomerular filtration rate marker. In this simplified representation of contrast agent elimination, the distribution phase (hatched area) is neglected, which leads to underestimation of the true area under the curve.

Non-radioactive compounds used to measure GFR include inulin and iohexol. The fructose polymer inulin (Mr ~ 5 kDa) satisfies the criteria as an ideal marker of GFR (although it should be noted that even inulin has some extra-renal clearance; equivalent to nearly 6 mL/min for a 70 kg human) and inulin clearance using a constant infusion urinary clearance approach has long been regarded as the gold standard measure of GFR. Acceptable single bolus plasma clearance approaches have also been evaluated. However, the lack of availability of simple laboratory methods of measurement remains an impediment to universal usage and, in practice, a variety of alternative, 'silver' standard estimates of GFR are used including iohexol, ^{125}I-iothalamate, ^{51}Cr-EDTA and ^{99m}Tc-diethylenetri-aminepentaacetic acid (DTPA).

Of these iohexol, an X-ray contrast agent, has the advantage that it is also non-radioisotopic, enabling analysis to be delayed and the procedure to be undertaken outside of nuclear medicine facilities. Single bolus plasma clearance of iohexol demonstrates excellent agreement with constant infusion urinary inulin clearance. Biological variability in patients with kidney disease using this technique is low (approximately 6%) and outpatient procedures based on filter paper blood spots have been described.

The radioisotopic techniques all have relative advantages and disadvantages. ^{99m}Tc-DTPA has the advantage that it can also be used for gamma camera imaging but it has been associated with problems of plasma protein binding of the tracer, although more recent formulations have minimised this. ^{125}I-iothalamate is no longer approved for intravascular use in some countries. ^{51}Cr-EDTA is generally preferred to ^{99m}Tc-DTPA and ^{125}I-iothalamate since its clearance is considered to be closest to that of inulin and the British Nuclear Medicine Society has endorsed its use as the standard clinical measure of GFR.

Measurement of GFR using endogenous substances

Although the clearance of infused markers is generally considered an accurate assessment of GFR, to date these procedures have generally been considered too costly and cumbersome for routine use. Creatinine and certain low molecular weight proteins (e.g. cystatin C) have been used as endogenous markers of GFR. The use of urea in this context is of limited value and will not be discussed further. Endogenous markers obviate the need for injection and require only a single blood sample, simplifying the procedure for the patient, clinician and laboratory.

CREATININE
The most widely used endogenous marker of GFR is creatinine, expressed either as its serum[a] concentration or its renal clearance. Creatinine is measured in virtually all clinical laboratories as a test of kidney function. Both chemical and enzymatic methods are used to measure creatinine in body fluids. Most laboratories use adaptations of the same assay for measurements in both serum and urine.

---

[a] creatinine measurements are equivalent in serum and plasma. We have used the term 'serum' throughout this chapter.

The use of creatinine as a marker of GFR was first developed in 1926 by Rehberg. Creatinine (Mr 113 Da) is freely filtered at the glomerulus and its concentration is inversely related to GFR. As a GFR marker it is convenient and cheap to measure but is affected by age, gender, exercise, certain drugs (e.g. cimetidine, trimethoprim), muscle mass and nutritional status. Creatine in muscle is converted to creatinine when meat is cooked with resultant increases in serum creatinine after cooked meat ingestion. Furthermore, a small (but significant) and variable proportion of the creatinine appearing in the urine is derived from tubular secretion; typically 7-10% is due to tubular secretion, but this is increased in the presence of renal insufficiency. Perhaps most importantly, serum creatinine concentration remains within the reference interval until significant renal function has been lost (Figure 3.7). Since serum creatinine is derived from creatine and phosphocreatine breakdown in muscle, the reference interval encompasses the range of muscle mass observed in the population. This contributes to the insensitivity of creatinine as a marker of diminished GFR. Additionally, in patients with CKD, extra-renal clearance of creatinine becomes significant due to degradation by bacterial overgrowth in the small intestine, further blunting the anticipated increase in serum creatinine in response to falling GFR. Consequently, serum creatinine measurement will not detect patients with stage 2 CKD and will also fail to identify many patients with stage 3 CKD. Thus, while an increased serum creatinine concentration does generally equate to impaired kidney function, a normal serum creatinine does not necessarily equate to normal kidney function. Because of all these limitations, it is recommended that serum creatinine measurement alone is not used to assess kidney function.

A method for the assay of serum creatinine was first described by Jaffe in 1886 (Figure 3.8). This involved the reaction of creatinine with alkaline sodium picrate to form an orange-red coloured complex. Most chemical methods for measuring creatinine are still based on this reaction although, more than one hundred years later, the reaction mechanism and the structure of the product remain unclear. Although there are now a variety of approaches to creatinine measurement, including enzymatic, high performance liquid chromatography (HPLC) and isotope dilution-mass spectrometry (ID-MS) methods, the Jaffe assay in either end-point or, more commonly, kinetic mode remains widely used. Measurement of creatinine using the Jaffe reaction suffers from three main problems: (1) non-specificity, (2) spectral interferences and (3) non-standardised calibration.

The relationship between serum creatinine and GFR

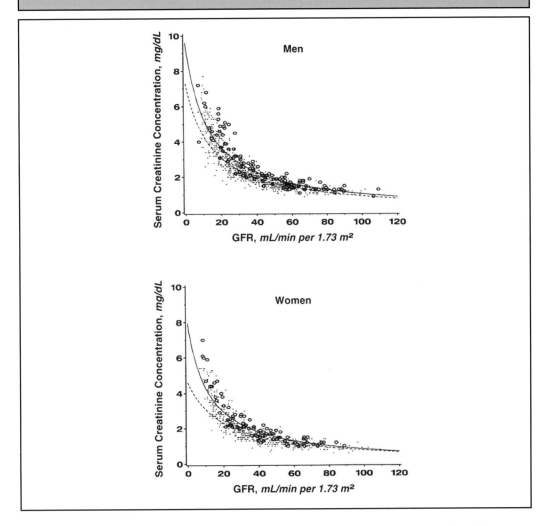

Figure 3.7. Relationship between serum creatinine and glomerular filtration rate (GFR). The figure illustrates the inverse curvilinear relationship between serum creatinine and GFR; that the relationship is different in men and women; and, that the relationship is different in Caucasians (dashed lines and dots) and Black-Americans (solid lines and circles). Each point represents the baseline measurement for one patient during the MDRD Study. GFR was measured as the renal clearance of ^{125}I-iothalamate. To convert mg/dL to µmol/L, multiply by 88.4. Reproduced with permission from Levey AS, Bosch JP, Lewis JB, Greene T, Rogers N, Roth D. A more accurate method to estimate glomerular filtration rate from serum creatinine: a new prediction equation. Modification of Diet in Renal Disease Study Group. Ann Intern Med 1999; **130**: 461-70.

Jaffe's original description of a creatinine assay

Ueber den Niederschlag, welchen Pikrinsäure in normalem Harn erzeugt und über eine neue Reaction des Kreatinins.

Von

M. Jaffe.

(Aus dem Laboratorium für medicin. Chemie zu Königsberg i. Pr.)
(Der Redaktion zugegangen am 26. Juni 1886.)

In der physiolog.-chemischen Literatur finden sich nur sehr spärliche Angaben über das Verhalten normalen Harns auf Zusatz von Prikrinsäure.

In K. B. Hofmann's Lehrbuch der Zoochemie heisst es S. 402: «Fügt man gesättigte Pikrinsäurelösung zu Menschenharn, so bleibt derselbe anfänglich klar, dann setzt sich (nach 3—4 Stunden) ein mässiger, gelbgefärbter, aus Harnsäurekrystallen und feinen Nadeln bestehender Bodensatz ab». H. Beaunis (Nouveaux éléments de Physiologie humaine) sagt S. 776: «l'acide picrique en precipite des cristaux d'acide urique» und H. Huppert in seiner Bearbeitung von Neubauer-Vogel's Analyse des Harns giebt S. 124 an, dass normaler Harn beim Kochen mit Pikrinsäure einen starken flockigen Niederschlag giebt.

Die gelegentliche Verwendung der Pikrinsäure zum Nachweise von Eiweissstoffen war für mich die Veranlassung die Erscheinungen, welche diese Säure in normalem Urin hervorruft, genauer zu verfolgen.

Es ergab sich Folgendes:

Wenn man menschlichen Harn mit conc. wässriger Pikrinsäurelösung versetzt, so bleibt er anfangs klar, scheidet aber im Laufe der nächsten Stunden meistens ein spärliches krystallinisches Sediment ab.

Review of the sedimentation process which is caused in normal urine by picric acid and a new reaction of creatinine

By M Jaffe

(From the Laboratory of Medical Chemistry in Koenigsberg, Prussia)
(Submitted to the editor on 26th June 1886)

In the physiological chemistry literature there is only very sparse information about the reaction of normal urine with picric acid.

In KB Hofmann's Textbook of Zoological Chemistry page 402 states "If saturated picric acid solution is added to human urine it will initially remain clear and after a period of 3 to 4 hours a yellow needle crystal sediment made of uric acid will form".

H Beaunis (New Elements of Human Physiology) states page 776: "Picric acid precipitates uric crystals" and H Huppert in his application of the new Bauer-Vogels' Analysis of Urine states on page 124, that normal urine when boiled with picric acid creates a strong cloudy flaky sediment.

The occasional use of picric acid for the identification of protein was the reason for me to investigate the reaction caused by the addition of this acid to urine.

The following was observed:

If human urine is titrated with concentrated picric acid solution it is initially clear, but over a period of the next hour a thin crystalline sediment forms.

Figure 3.8 Jaffe's original description of an assay for measuring creatinine. We are grateful to Mr Mark Vickery for the translation into English.

The Jaffe reaction is not specific for creatinine. Many compounds have been reported to produce a Jaffe-like chromogen, including protein, glucose, ascorbic acid, ketone bodies, pyruvate, guanidine, blood-substitute products and cephalosporins. The degree of interference from these compounds varies both between patients and with the precise reaction conditions of the assay. Jaffe assays are also highly susceptible to spectral interference from bilirubin, haemoglobin and lipaemia. Enzymatic assays are not immune to these effects either. Problems of both bias and imprecision with creatinine measurement remain and, in both cases, have their greatest impact in the near-normal range. Between laboratory variation (coefficient of variation) across the UK is currently approximately 5% at a concentration of 120 μmol/L and there is significant bias between method groups. Much of the between laboratory difference is due to calibration differences. Hitherto there has been a lack of a universally accepted creatinine standard.

Some manufacturers have attempted partially to address these problems by aligning the calibration of their assays so that results more closely mimic those of the reference method (ID-MS). The aim of this is to account for reaction of Jaffe-based methods with non-creatinine chromogens. These so-called 'compensated' assays produce lower results at concentrations within the reference range, but they make an assumption that the non-creatinine chromogen interference is constant between samples, which is clearly an over-simplification. A working group of the International Federation of Clinical Chemistry has recently addressed this issue through the preparation of a standardised reference material (SRM) 967. This measure should improve inter-laboratory agreement in creatinine measurement, but will still not eliminate problems due to the variable non-specificity of Jaffe reactions. Such problems can only be overcome by the use of more specific methods, i.e. enzymatic assays for routine clinical purposes. Increasingly, serum creatinine measurements are being used to generate estimates of GFR using equations (see below). Inter-laboratory differences in creatinine bias and specificity is an area that the laboratory community urgently needs to resolve.

CREATININE CLEARANCE

Popper and Mandel in 1937 were the first to develop the use of endogenous creatinine clearance. Because creatinine is endogenously produced and released into body fluids at a constant rate, its clearance can be measured as an indicator of GFR. Creatinine clearance has in the past been seen as more sensitive for detection of renal dysfunction than serum creatinine measurement. However, it requires a timed urine collection, which introduces its own inaccuracies, and is inconvenient and unpleasant. In adults, the intra-individual day-to-day coefficient of variation for repeated measures of creatinine clearance exceeds 25%. Although tubular secretion undermines the theoretical value of creatinine as a marker of GFR, in the context of creatinine clearance this has previously to some extent been offset by the use of non-specific Jaffe methods to measure serum creatinine, which lead to an overestimation of serum concentration (see above). Nevertheless, creatinine clearance usually equals or exceeds inulin GFR in adults by a factor of 10-40% at clearances above 80 mL/min. However, as GFR falls, tubular secretion of creatinine rises proportionately and the creatinine clearance can reach nearly twice that of inulin. Tubular reabsorption of creatinine has also been reported at low GFRs but may represent diffusion of creatinine through gap junctions between tubular cells or directly through the tubular epithelial cells, down a concentration gradient. Whatever the mechanism, this further devalues the use of creatinine clearance. Hence, at best, creatinine clearance can only provide a crude index of GFR.

ESTIMATED GFR

The mathematical relationship between serum creatinine and GFR can be improved by correcting for the confounding variables that make that relationship non-linear. More than 25 different equations have been derived that estimate GFR using serum creatinine corrected for some or all of gender, body size, race and age. These may produce a better estimate of GFR than serum creatinine alone. Indeed, the UK NSF for Renal Disease and the National Kidney Foundation of the USA, in addition to other international organisations, have recommended that such estimates should be used in preference to serum creatinine. The Cockcroft and Gault and MDRD Study equations have been widely used in adults. Two further equations (Schwartz and Counahan-Barratt) are recommended for use in children (see below).

The Cockcroft and Gault equation is one of the earliest, and most widely used, of these equations. The authors published their formula in 1976 using data from 236 hospital inpatients who had two creatinine clearance determinations which differed by less than 20% from each other. The ethnic origin of these subjects was not stated, but it is highly likely that most, if not all, subjects were Caucasian. The mean of the two serum creatinine and creatinine clearance estimations was used in deriving their formula using regression analysis, taking age and weight into consideration. Creatinine was measured using the Jaffe reaction (Technicon Autoanalyser method N-11B) and the authors reported that non-creatinine chromogens would be expected to interfere in this assay. A 15% reduction was recommended when applying the formula to women, although no evidence was given to support this factor.

Creatinine clearance (mL/min) = [(140 - age (years)) x weight (kg)/(0.814 x plasma creatinine (μmol/L)] x (0.85 if female)

The observed correlation coefficient between their predicted creatinine clearance and measured creatinine clearance was 0.83 (R^2 0.69), with predicted and mean measured clearance values differing by 20% or less in 67% of patients.

The 6-variable (6-v) MDRD equation was published in 1999 following a retrospective re-analysis of the MDRD Study, which has been described in Chapter 2. GFR was determined in 1628 predominantly middle-aged patients with known kidney disease using ^{125}I-iothalamate and expressed per 1.73 m² BSA. Creatinine was measured in a central laboratory using a kinetic Jaffe assay on a Beckman Astra CX3 analyser. Stepwise multiple regression modelling on log-transformed data was used to determine the set of variables that best predicted GFR. The inclusion of serum urea and albumin concentrations was found to improve the predictive strength of the model.

GFR (mL/min/1.73 m^2) = 170 x [serum creatinine (µmol/L) x 0.011312]$^{-0.999}$ x [age]$^{-0.176}$ x [0.762 if patient is female] x [1.180 if patient is black] x [serum urea (mmol/L) x 2.801]$^{-0.170}$ x [serum albumin (g/L) x 0.1]$^{+0.318}$

The lack of requirement of knowledge of body weight was a practical advantage compared to the Cockcroft and Gault equation, which also gave poorer accuracy in their hands. The requirement for measurement of albumin and urea in addition to creatinine was clearly a limitation of the 6-v MDRD equation, increasing both analytical costs and the contribution of analytical variation. Recognising this, in 2000 these workers subsequently published an abbreviated (4-variable, 4-v) version of the equation, which does not require these measurements and did not result in appreciable loss of accuracy (R^2 0.892 against ^{125}I-iothalamate GFR), with 90% of subjects having a GFR estimate within 30% of the measured value.

GFR (mL/min/1.73 m^2) = 186 x [serum creatinine (µmol/L) x 0.011312]$^{-1.154}$ x [age]$^{-0.203}$ x [1.212 if black] x [0.742 if female]

The 4-v MDRD equation has several advantages compared to the Cockcroft and Gault equation: it was developed and validated in a large population; there is no requirement for patient weight; the validation was against an iothalamate clearance estimate of GFR and reported GFR is corrected for BSA. Unlike the Cockcroft and Gault equation, the model also takes into account the fact that the relationship between serum creatinine and GFR differs between Caucasians and African-Americans. Since its publication, a series of studies have compared the applicability of the Cockcroft and Gault and 4-v MDRD equations in a variety of clinical settings. From these, a general conclusion can be drawn that, for the detection of patients with stage 3-5 CKD, the MDRD equation provides a more accurate, and clinically acceptable, assessment of GFR than the Cockcroft and Gault equation. Both equations demonstrate deteriorating performance as GFR increases; however, it must be remembered that a diagnosis of stage 2 CKD is not based upon GFR alone, but requires other supporting evidence of kidney disease, most notably proteinuria or microalbuminuria. Neither equation adequately estimates GFR in patients with physiological range GFRs, an important consideration when monitoring patients with diabetes or assessing the suitability of potential kidney donors (Figure 3.9).

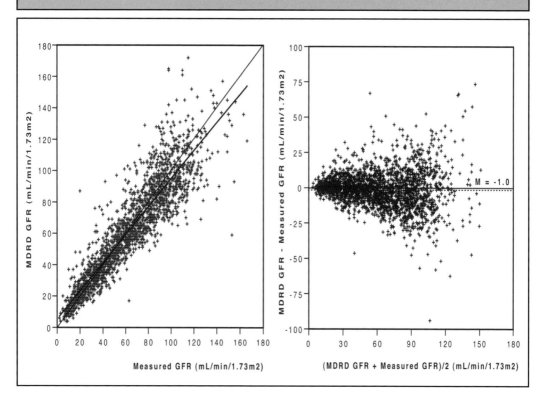

Performance of MDRD Study formula for GFR

Figure 3.9. Performance of the Modification of Diet in Renal Disease (MDRD) Study formula as an estimate of measured glomerular filtration rate (GFR). The data are illustrated as a scatter plot (left panel) and a Bland and Altman plot (right panel). The mean difference (M) is represented by the dashed line. GFR was measured using a ^{51}Cr-EDTA technique. Reproduced with permission from Froissart M, Rossert J, Jacquot C, Paillard M, Houillier P. Predictive performance of the modification of diet in renal disease and Cockcroft-Gault equations for estimating renal function. J Am Soc Nephrol 2005; **16**: 763-773.

Inter-laboratory differences in creatinine measurement have been discussed above. These differences, compounded by poor precision around the upper limit of the reference interval, can have a significant impact on the estimation of GFR using these equation-based approaches, such that patients may or may not be diagnosed as having stage 3 CKD dependent upon the laboratory undertaking the analysis. Furthermore, the MDRD equation is anchored to a non-specific kinetic rate assay for creatinine on an analytical platform that will not be available in perpetuity. Recognising this, in 2005 the authors of the MDRD study published a re-analysis of their data enabling the MDRD equation to be anchored to an ID-MS creatinine assay. In this version of the 4-v MDRD equation the constant factor 186 is replaced with the constant 175. In England, the Department of Health has recommended that this version of the equation should be implemented by laboratories to enable estimation of GFR. External quality assessment schemes can provide correction factors enabling different creatinine assays to be linked to the reference ID-MS method, thus improving inter-laboratory agreement in respect of GFR estimation.

There are several clinical situations in which precise knowledge of GFR is important, and where reliance on equation-based estimates of GFR should be avoided. These include cancer chemotherapy, or the use of any other drug that is renally excreted and has a narrow therapeutic margin; the assessment of potential living related kidney donors; and the assessment of GFR in patients with muscle wasting disorders, including spina bifida and paraplegia. When accurate GFR information is required, reference methods should be used; for potential living kidney donors, use of a radioisotopic estimate of GFR, preferably combined with gamma-camera imaging to assess differential kidney function, is recommended by the British Transplantation Society.

Serum creatinine is an imperfect marker of GFR and therefore it is not altogether surprising that equations based predominantly upon it are imperfect. Their use cannot circumvent the very significant spectral interferences affecting serum creatinine measurement and the equations are critically susceptible to variations in creatinine assay calibration and specificity. Recently, the significant negative impact of cooked meat ingestion on estimated GFR has also been appreciated. However, despite these major limitations, the use of estimates of GFR has been shown to improve the recognition of patients with CKD, compared to use of serum creatinine alone. Internationally, recommendations now generally favour use of the 4-v MDRD equation for estimating GFR in adults.

CYSTATIN C (AND OTHER LOW MOLECULAR WEIGHT PROTEINS)
A number of proteins with molecular weights of less than 30 kDa are predominantly cleared from the circulation by renal filtration and can be considered to be relatively freely filtered at the glomerular filtration barrier. These include β_2-microglobulin, RBP, α_1-microglobulin, and cystatin C. These proteins are filtered at the glomerulus, then reabsorbed (and metabolised) in the proximal tubule or excreted into the urine, and thus they are entirely eliminated from the circulation. Therefore, they have the potential to meet the criteria for use as a marker of GFR. The most promising of these is cystatin C; all the other proteins have been shown to have serum concentrations that are influenced by non-renal factors such as inflammation and liver disease. The relationship between the circulating concen-

tration of cystatin C shows the same curvilinear form as serum creatinine, but several groups have demonstrated that its measurement may offer a more sensitive and specific means of monitoring changes in GFR than serum creatinine.

Cystatin C is a low molecular weight (Mr 12.8 kDa) protein synthesised by all nucleated cells, where its physiological role is that of a cysteine protease inhibitor. With regard to renal function, its most important attributes are its small size and high pI (9.2), which enable it to be more freely filtered than the above mentioned proteins at the glomerulus. The gene has been sequenced and the promotor region has been identified as a housekeeping type, with no known regulatory elements. Consequently, the production rate of cystatin C has always been considered to be constant, although several recent publications suggest an influence of thyroid hormones. Serum concentrations of cystatin C appear to be unaffected by muscle mass, diet or gender. There are no known extra-renal routes of elimination, with clearance from the circulation only by glomerular filtration.

Cystatin C has mainly been measured using precise latex particle-enhanced turbidimetric or nephelometric immunoassays. Measurement of cystatin C appears resistant to the spectral interferences affecting creatinine assays. There are a number of reports documenting the correlation between serum cystatin C and creatinine (as a reciprocal), and GFR as assessed by ^{51}Cr-EDTA or other exogenous marker clearance. In almost all cases, the correlation with cystatin C is superior to that with creatinine. Furthermore, cystatin C concentration increases sooner than that of creatinine as GFR declines (at approximately 60 mL/min/1.73 m^2 compared to about 40 mL/min/1.73 m^2 for serum creatinine). Cystatin C is therefore especially useful when trying to detect mild impairment of kidney function.

Kidney function assessment at the extremes of age
At birth, serum creatinine concentrations approximate those of the maternal circulation. Serum creatinine concentrations fall rapidly during the neonatal period, with slower falls being observed in premature infants. Serum creatinine concentrations are lower in infants than in adults, despite their lower GFR, reflecting the lower muscle mass (decreased creatinine production rate). In the setting of paediatric intensive care medicine, the usefulness of serum creatinine may be further limited by analytical interferences due to high concentrations of bilirubin and competition with creatinine for tubular secretion by commonly used drugs (e.g. trimethoprim, cimetidine).

Because of these difficulties, two creatinine-based formulae, proposed in 1976 by Counahan *et al* (the Counahan-Barratt formula) and Schwartz *et al*, have been widely used to predict GFR in children.

Counahan-Barratt formula:

GFR (mL/min/1.73 m^2) = 38 x length (cm)/serum creatinine (µmol/L)

Schwartz formula:

GFR (mL/min/1.73 m^2) = 49 x length (cm) /serum creatinine (µmol/L)

Both formulae require measurement of body length/height, as height is proportional to muscle mass; differences in the constant between the formulae probably reflect methodological differences in the original studies (e.g. creatinine assay differences or use of different gold standards for GFR estimation). Both formulae provide an improved estimate of kidney function compared to serum creatinine alone or creatinine clearance, although both are also imprecise. Studies describing the accuracy of the estimate show that approximately 75% of Schwartz formula estimates of GFR are within 30% of the measured GFR by inulin clearance. Comparable studies of the Counahan-Barratt formula show that 70% to 86% of estimates fall within 30% of GFR measured by ^{51}Cr-EDTA. The Schwartz formula has been shown to overestimate GFR compared to inulin clearance, the bias increasing with decreasing GFR. In the UK, paediatric nephrologists tend to favour the Schwartz formula.

Serum cystatin C concentrations in infants appear to reflect GFR more closely than serum creatinine, being increased in the first three months of life and then falling to approximate adult concentrations by age one year. Further, the diagnostic accuracy of cystatin C for reduced GFR is superior to that of creatinine in children.

Serum creatinine concentrations in healthy older people are not dissimilar to those in younger people, except in nonagenarians and centenarians, despite the decrease in GFR that occurs, on average, with ageing (see Chapter 1). Possible reasons for this include reduced muscle mass and poorer nutrition. Whatever the reason, the same serum creatinine concentration may indicate very different degrees of kidney function in younger and older people, and a normal concentration cannot exclude significant renal impairment. The effects of this may be marked and are commonly not appreciated. Several studies have suggested that serum cystatin C does reflect the age-related decline in kidney function and appears to be more sensitive than serum creatinine for detection of reduced GFR in older people.

Further reading

URINARY EXAMINATION
Simmerville JA, Maxted WC, Pahira JJ. Urinalysis: a comprehensive review. Am Family Physician 2005; **71**: 1153-62.

PROTEINURIA
Beetham R, Cattell WR. Proteinuria: pathophysiology, significance and recommendations for measurement in clinical practice. Ann Clin Biochem 1993; **30**: 425-434.

D'Amico G, Bazzi C. Pathophysiology of proteinuria. Kidney Int 2003; **63**: 809-825.

ALBUMINURIA
National Institute for Health and Clinical Excellence, Management of type 2 diabetes (update) CG66. Clinical Guideline May 2008.
www.nice.org.uk/GuidanceCG66/NICEguidance/pdf/English
Accessed: December 2008.

Newman DJ, Mattock MB, Dawnay ABS, Kerry S, McGuire A, Yaqoob M, Hitman GA, Hawke C. Systematic review on urine albumin testing for early detection of diabetic complications. Health Technol Assess 2005; **9** (30).

GLOMERULAR FILTRATION RATE
Lamb EJ, Tomson CRV, Roderick PJ. Estimating kidney function in adults using formulae. Ann Clin Biochem 2005; **42**: 321-345.

Levey AS, Coresh J, Greene T, *et al.* Expressing the Modification of Diet in Renal Disease Study equation for estimating glomerular filtration rate with standardized serum creatinine values. Clin Chem 2007; **53**: 766-772.

CREATININE
Perrone RD, Madias NE, Levey AS. Serum creatinine as an index of renal function: New insights into old concepts. Clin Chem 1992; **38**: 1933-1953.

CYSTATIN C
Laterza OF, Price CP, Scott MG. Cystatin C: an improved estimator of glomerular filtration rate? Clin Chem 2002; **48**: 699-707.

Newman DJ. Cystatin C. Ann Clin Biochem 2002; **39**: 89-104.

Effects of ageing on kidney function tests

Lamb EJ, O'Riordan SE, Delaney MP. Ageing and the kidney: pathology, assessment and management. Clin Chim Acta 2003; **334:** 25-40.

Chapter 4

Acute renal failure

Introduction

Acute renal failure (ARF, more recently called 'acute kidney injury') describes a clinical scenario of kidney failure that develops over hours or days rather than weeks and months. ARF can often be superimposed on established CKD and is then referred to as 'acute on chronic' renal failure. The aetiology of ARF is traditionally separated into three major groups: pre-renal, renal and post-renal causes. This schema is useful since it allows the clinician to focus on the appropriate investigations to be performed in a logical order. The diagnosis is first considered upon receipt of laboratory investigations that reveal increases in serum concentrations of urea and creatinine. It is important to recognise ARF early as appropriate treatment can be life saving and renal recovery will often ensue. ARF is a common medical emergency with a significant mortality.

There are difficulties in assessing the incidence, prevalence and risk factors for the development of ARF. An extensive literature has evolved that has assessed the relative merits of predicting those patients at risk of developing ARF whilst in hospital. However, the interpretation of the data is limited since the populations tested and the criteria used to define ARF are heterogeneous. Currently, there is no standard or unifying definition in clinical or research practice. This leads to difficulties when comparing approaches to predictors of ARF and in terms of clinical interventions. For example, ARF may be defined as a rise in the serum creatinine concentration by an arbitrary percentage or reaching an arbitrary absolute number. Alternative definitions of ARF may include development of reduced urine volume (< 400 mL/24 h), referred to as oliguria, or the need for RRT in the form of dialysis. Caution is also required when interpreting measurements of serum creatinine concentration in ARF, since creatinine concentration may decrease as a result of dilution following intravenous fluid replacement and creatinine concentration only rises above the reference range when there has been a significant fall in GFR leading to an under-estimate of the true incidence of ARF. Classification systems based on the combination of susceptibility (includes pre-existing CKD and the presence of another risk factor such as diabetes), nature and timing of insult, biomarker response, urine output and end-organ consequences have been proposed. For example, the RIFLE classification (named by the severity of renal impairment: Risk, Injury, Failure, Loss, End-stage kidney disease) has been demonstrated to be a valuable method to evaluate ARF after cardiac surgery, with patients in the severe category having a higher 90-day mortality rate.

Nevertheless, population studies that utilise laboratory databases have suggested an annual incidence of ARF of 80-140 per million population (pmp) per year with approximately 50% of these requiring dialysis. Older people are particularly at risk. It is estimated that ARF develops in 5% of patients admitted to hospital and a prospective study of the initial hospital management of ARF confirmed that in almost 40% of cases ARF was iatrogenic or preventable. The survival of patients who develop ARF in the setting of multiple organ failure is poor, although patients with single organ failure have a relatively good prognosis. Many patients with complex medical diseases and significant co-morbidities are now referred to renal unit programmes for assessment and treatment. The overall survival of patients with ARF has changed very little over the past two decades. The outcome may be skewed by the fact that more elderly patients and those with greater co-morbidity are treated for ARF. Approximately 90% of patients with isolated ARF requiring RRT should survive to hospital discharge. However, if there is combined severe acute renal and respiratory failure, the survival drops to 45%, and in multi-organ failure, only 5-15% of patients survive to discharge. Following major surgery, ARF occurs in 1-10 % of patients. Patients who develop ARF have higher rates of mortality and resource utilisation, with the worst values in those that require RRT. Even small changes in serum creatinine concentration after cardiac surgery are associated with mortality; there is also an association with increased long-term mortality.

Causes of ARF

Classification

The classic method for categorising the causes of ARF depends on a system that identifies whether the insult to kidney function occurs before the kidneys (pre-renal), occurs within the kidneys (renal) or occurs as a result of mechanical obstruction to flow of urine away from the kidneys via the ureters and bladder (post-renal) (Figure 4.1). Pre-renal ARF implies some form of relative hypoperfusion of the kidneys which may be a result of dehydration, haemorrhage or any other cause of cardiovascular collapse. Pre-renal ARF can be considered to be an appropriate physiological response to hypovolaemia, resulting in intense renal conservation of sodium and water at the expense of GFR. Pre-renal ARF can be treated and reversed quickly with appropriate measures to restore the circulation and renal perfusion. However, prolonged renal ischaemia may cause tubular cellular damage that persists despite correction of the original insult. This is referred to as acute tubular necrosis (ATN*) and can be considered to be the commonest 'renal' cause of ARF, as described below.

*The term 'ATN' is somewhat misleading insofar as necrosis *per se* is seldom seen, rather tubular damage.

Causes of acute renal failure (ARF)

Type	Lesion	Cause
Pre-renal ARF		Dehydration Haemorrhage Diarrhoea Post-operative fluid and blood losses Sepsis Acute cardiac failure Aortic dissection
Intrinsic renal disease	Glomerular disease	Rapidly progressive glomerulonephritis ANCA-associated vasculitides Goodpasture's disease Systemic lupus erythematosus Crescentic lesions complicating glomerular disease Cryoglobulinaemia Post-infectious glomerulonephritis
	Tubulointerstitial disease	Any pre-renal cause leading to ATN (the most common cause of ARF) Drug nephrotoxicity (non-steroidal anti-inflammatory drugs [NSAIDs], ACE inhibitors, aminoglycoside antibiotics, amphotericin) Allergic tubulo-interstitial nephritis associated with antibiotics and NSAIDs Sarcoidosis Pyelonephritis Myeloma cast nephropathy
	Microvascular disease	Thrombotic microangiopathies (haemolytic-uraemic syndrome/thrombotic thrombocytopaenic purpura, pre-eclamptic toxaemia, scleroderma)
	Miscellaneous	Contrast nephropathy Poisoning (e.g. methanol) Rhabdomyolysis Urate nephropathy Hepatorenal syndrome Cholesterol embolism Renal vein thrombosis
Post-renal ARF	Bladder outflow obstruction Bilateral renal calculi or calculi within a single kidney Retroperitoneal fibrosis	Benign and malignant prostate disease Invasive bladder carcinoma

Figure 4.1 Causes of acute renal failure (ARF)

In addition to ATN, intrinsic kidney diseases affecting glomerular function, interstitial nephritis or blood vessel damage may cause 'renal' or parenchymal ARF. These diseases should be considered in the setting of ARF that has not responded to primary fluid resuscitation, particularly if there is haematuria and proteinuria in the absence of urinary tract obstruction. Supporting laboratory evidence may be available and a kidney biopsy can be performed to confirm the underlying diagnosis in selected cases.

Obstruction of the urinary tract is a common cause of post-renal kidney failure. It is particularly common in older men due to prostatic hypertrophy leading to bladder outflow obstruction. Other causes include invasive bladder cancer, other pelvic malignancies, renal stone disease and retroperitoneal fibrosis. Urinary tract dilatation is readily diagnosed non-invasively on ultrasound scanning and is indicative of obstruction.

Acute tubular necrosis
Intrinsic ARF can be caused by primary vascular, glomerular, or interstitial disorders. However, as indicated above, the underlying renal parenchymal lesion in the majority of cases is ATN, caused by ischaemic or nephrotoxic insults. In 50% of cases of hospital-acquired ARF, the cause is multifactorial. The kidneys are particularly vulnerable to ischaemia. Blood flow through the kidneys is approximately 20-25% of the total cardiac output, i.e. 1.1 L/minute, with the majority (> 90%) through the renal cortex. The deeper blood vessels, known as the vasa rectae, allow oxygen to perfuse freely across their walls. In the normal kidney, the cortex is well oxygenated with a pO_2 of 9 kPa. Conversely, the outer medulla is relatively hypoxic with a pO_2 of 3 kPa, as a result of the counter-current mechanism in the vasa rectae and increased oxygen extraction and consumption by the cells of the thick ascending limb of the loop of Henle, particularly at the corticomedullary junction. The metabolic demands of the tubular epithelial cells are substantial, since they depend on Na^+-K^+-ATPase for normal function. As a consequence of their high ATP demands in a region of relative hypoxia, tubular epithelial cells are prone to injury following renal ischaemia.

Oliguria is a physiological response to renal hypoperfusion. The renal circulation is capable of autoregulation, i.e. it is able to maintain relatively constant blood flow over changes in mean arterial pressure in the range of 80-180 mmHg, equivalent to systolic/diastolic blood pressure readings in the range between 90/70 mmHg and 260/140mm Hg. Autoregulation will fail outside these limits. The physiological renal response to volume depletion is initially afferent arteriolar vasodilatation and efferent arteriolar vasoconstriction to maintain glomerular filtration pressure. Under normal conditions, intra-renal blood flow and GFR are tightly autoregulated by a complex system of vasoactive mediators and auto-

nomic activity. If this autoregulation fails there is intense and persistent vasoconstriction of renal vessels leading to ischaemic renal injury.

PATHOPHYSIOLOGY OF ATN.
Tubular cell injury occurs as a result of several processes acting simultaneously
(Figure 4.2).

Pathophysiology of acute tubular necrosis

MICROVASCULAR

Vasoconstriction *in response*
to:
endothelin, adenosine, angiotensin
II, thromboxane A2, leukotrienes,
sympathetic nerve activity

Vasodilation *in response* to:
nitric oxide, prostaglandin E2,
acetylcholine, bradykinin

Endothelial and vascular
smooth muscle cell structural
damage

Leucocyte-endothelial
adhesion, vascular obstruction,
leucocyte activation and
inflammation

O$_2$

Inflammatory
and vasoactive
mediators

TUBULAR

Cytoskeletal breakdown

Loss of polarity

Apoptosis and necrosis

Desquamation of viable
and necrotic cells

Tubular obstruction

Backleak

Figure 4.2 Pathophysiology of ischaemic acute renal failure
Reproduced with permission from Bonventre JV, Weinberg JM. Recent advances
in the pathophysiology of ischemic acute renal failure. J Am Soc Nephrol 2003; **14:**
2199-2210.

1) *Vasoconstriction.* The interactions of mediators that cause intense vasoconstriction in patients at risk of ARF due to ATN are not known. Prolonged vasoconstriction occurs in experimental models seen long after the initial stimulus. This
prolongs renal injury and delays recovery. Possible mechanisms involve endothe-
lins (e.g. ET1 is a potent vasoconstrictor), nitric oxide (vasodilator, reduced
endothelial production in renal ischaemia), AII (a potent vasoconstrictor), catecholamines and adenosine.

2) *Tubuloglomerular feedback.* The macula densa is the area of the nephron represented by tall columnar epithelium in the last section of the thick ascending loop of Henle, before the distal tubule, as the tubule lies against its contiguous glomerular tuft and is in communication with the JGA of the afferent arteriole. The cells of the JGA contain renin and are under sympathetic tone (Chapter 1). Decreased perfusion leads to reduced stretch in the afferent arterioles which increases renin secretion via local and neurohumoral mechanisms. Glomerular filtration is also affected by activation of tubuloglomerular feedback. In the normal state tubuloglomerular feedback acts as a negative feedback system. If mean arterial pressure is increased, and GFR rises, the increased delivery of sodium and chloride ions to the macula densa leads to a reduction in GFR through vasopressor effects on the afferent arteriole. The mediators of this effect are thought to be adenosine, prostaglandins and AII. During a period of hypoperfusion, autoregulatory mechanisms ensure avid absorption of sodium and water by the proximal tubule and reduced sodium and chloride delivery to the distal part of the nephron. The cells of the macula densa are sensitive to decreased chloride ion concentration and mediators promote renin secretion from the juxtaglomerular cells to maintain the GFR via AII-mediated effects. However, with prolonged hypoperfusion and tissue ischaemia the proximal tubule cells become damaged. There is increased delivery of sodium and chloride ions to the distal nephron and the macula densa responds by mediating a further decrease in GFR via tubuloglomerular feedback. The ability of the macula densa to decrease the GFR when distal delivery is enhanced prevents distal reabsorptive capacity from being overwhelmed, which could lead to potentially life threatening losses of sodium and water. Viewed in this light, it may be macula densa flow that is being maintained by autoregulation and tubuloglomerular feedback. Thus the reduction in GFR, which is not easily explained by any histological abnormalities, may in part represent an appropriate tubuloglomerular feedback response to maintain sodium balance.

3) *Hypoxia within the corticomedullary junction.* The tubular cells are very susceptible to ischaemic necrosis compared with glomerular cells due to the relatively hypoxic renal medulla. The straight segment of the proximal tubule (S3) is the most sensitive to injury due to relative hypoxia of the region in which these segments lie. Ischaemia disrupts the actin cytoskeleton with loss of polarity of the cell and translocation of Na^+-K^+-ATPase from the basal membrane to the apical (luminal) membrane. Sodium is pumped into the cell and causes swelling and death.

4) *Obstruction of the tubule.* Shedding of tubular cells and casts increases tubular pressure and disrupts the tubular basement membrane causing back-leakage of glomerular filtrate into the interstitium and venous system. This is referred to as

backfiltration and accounts for up to 40% of the observed reduction of the GFR in oliguria.

5) *Vascular congestion.* Congestion of intra-renal blood vessels causes a further reduction in the GFR. Activation and release of cytokines leads to aggregation of leucocytes, erythrocytes and platelets, resulting in congestion and vasoconstriction.

The characteristic lesions of ATN on microscopy include flattening of proximal tubule cell microvilli, epithelial cell flattening, and obstruction of the tubule lumen by shed epithelial cells and precipitated proteins. Following injury, the kidney undergoes repair with regeneration of tubular epithelium and restoration of glomerular haemodynamics. The medullary concentrating ability reappears slowly and the urine output increases; the patient often then enters a polyuric phase, with potential for excess urinary loss of electrolytes and water.

Despite an extensive literature suggesting that enhanced vasoconstriction is a fundamental contributor to the pathophysiology of ischaemic ARF, no vasodilator has been found to be useful in the prevention or treatment of ARF associated with ATN in man. Examples of those tested include low dose dopamine and ANP. This may in part be due to the fact that in many cases of ARF, there is underlying kidney damage, particularly in older people or patients with diabetes and hypertension, that is not necessarily identified by the serum creatinine concentration.

Clinical features of ARF

Although there are many potential causes of ARF, the clinical consequences of developing ARF share common pathways. ARF develops rapidly, and therefore the clinical picture is one of rapid electrolyte, acid-base and fluid imbalances that can be difficult to control. Oliguria, a reduction in urine output to less than that required to maintain physiological homeostasis, equates to a urine output of < 400 mL/24 h. In response to reduced glomerular filtration and the development of oliguria, the blood urea, creatinine and potassium concentrations will rise and severe metabolic acidosis may develop. To help to differentiate between acute and acute on chronic renal failure a biochemical history should be sought. This may involve investigation of the hospital laboratory database or telephone calls to other hospitals or primary care clinicians to obtain previous serum creatinine results.

Following a detailed history and examination to try to identify and remedy the cause of ARF, the priority of treatment is fluid resuscitation and correction of life threatening metabolic derangements. An attempt should be made to obtain a urine specimen for dipstick analysis (see below), microscopy and culture. Fluid balance charts should be established to monitor fluid input and loss, including both urinary and extra-renal losses. Fluid resuscitation can usually be performed with crystalloids such as 0.9% saline (normal saline). This solution is cheap and safe, but rapidly distributes to the extravascular spaces, resulting in oedema. Colloids such as modified gelatins, hydroxyethyl starch and albumin may remain in the vascular space for longer than crystalloid solutions. Meta-analysis comparing synthetic colloids with crystalloids has concluded that there is no proven benefit of colloids. Fluid replacement requirements need careful monitoring and review of the patient, with the emphasis on restoring an optimal circulatory volume without developing signs of fluid overload such as pulmonary oedema. Additional monitoring may include use of a central venous pressure (CVP) line. The insertion of a CVP line is a specialist skill requiring cannulation of the internal jugular vein, ideally utilising ultrasonic guidance facilities. However, where hypovolaemia is clinically apparent, the priority is to resuscitate the patient with fluid rather than delay treatment by establishing invasive monitoring. When the clinical assessment of circulating volume is unclear, invasive monitoring may be helpful to assess circulating volume, guide fluid replacement and provide access for drug administration. The target central venous pressure is 8-12 cm H_2O. A series of CVP measurements is useful to check the response to fluids.

Initial investigations in ARF

Urine dipstick testing is mandatory in all cases of ARF. Dipstick tests for blood and protein are positive in rapidly progressive glomerulonephritis and should prompt further investigation. Red blood cell casts on microscopy are suggestive of glomerular bleeding and are a feature of glomerular disease. A normal urine dipstick test may be seen in pre-renal ARF, ATN and obstruction.

Urinary electrolytes are seldom required or useful in the investigation of ARF. Measurement of urinary sodium excretion or fractional excretion of sodium attempts to differentiate 'pre-renal' ARF from established ATN. Tubular reabsorption of sodium with minimal excretion of sodium may be present in pre-renal ARF. High urine osmolality suggests that tubules are responding appropriately to ADH and retaining water avidly. In contrast, ATN is suggested by high sodium losses and lower osmolality as a result of tubular damage. Misleading results may be obtained in those patients taking diuretics since these drugs increase urinary sodium excretion. In practice the treatment of pre-renal ARF and ATN requires prompt and continued correction of hypovolaemia, so the urinary findings are not generally helpful (Figure 4.3).

Urinary electrolytes in pre-renal ARF and ATN

	Pre-renal	ATN
Urine sodium (mmol/L)	< 20	> 40
Urine osmolality (mmol/kg)	> 500	< 350
Fractional excretion of sodium % (FENa)*	< 1	> 2

These indices are of limited value as intermediate values are common and can be influenced by diuretic use and pre-existing tubular damage. As highlighted in the text the initial treatment of fluid replacement is the same for both groups.

*Urinary sodium excretion can be expressed as the fractional excretion of sodium (FENa) which relates sodium excretion to creatinine excretion and can be calculated by the equation:

FENa = sodium clearance/creatinine clearance

= $\dfrac{\text{Urine sodium x serum creatinine (mmol/L)}}{\text{Serum sodium x urine creatinine (mmol/L)}} \times 100$

Figure 4.3 Urinary electrolytes in pre-renal ARF and acute tubular necrosis

Laboratory testing of blood is crucial to the management of ARF. The clinical biochemistry laboratory is particularly important since regular testing of kidney function, electrolytes and acid-base balance is central to monitoring the severity of ARF as well as response to interventions. Blood tests also aid with establishing the underlying diagnosis where specific investigations are requested. An 'acute renal screen' should remain clearly focused on the most likely diagnoses. Suggested investigations are shown in Figure 4.4. Recovery from ATN is heralded by a polyuric phase of urine production as glomerular function recovers before tubular function. Polyuria recedes after a few days to weeks, but careful monitoring of serum creatinine and electrolyte concentrations is required to enable suitable fluid and electrolyte replacement. If the patient survives, recovery will usually occur within days or weeks following the removal of the initiating event.

Laboratory investigation of acute renal failure

Test	Indication/abnormality
Urine testing	
Urine dipstick	Haematuria and proteinuria suggests glomerular disease
Red cell casts on microscopy	Glomerular disease
Mid-stream urine for microscopy, culture and sensitivity	Urinary tract infection
Bence Jones protein	Monoclonal light chain mediated disease
Blood tests	
Serial electrolytes, creatinine and urea, including review of historical reports	Identify kidney failure
Venous plasma bicarbonate	Acidosis
Arterial blood gases	Metabolic acidosis
C-reactive protein	Inflammation and infection
Creatine kinase	Rhabdomyolysis
Calcium	↑ calcium - myeloma, hyperparathyroidism, sarcoidosis, malignancy, renal stones, iatrogenic ↓ calcium - advanced CKD, rhabdomyolysis
Phosphate	↑ phosphate - rhabdomyolysis, advanced CKD
Liver function tests	Suspected multi-organ involvement or abnormal coagulation
Albumin	Suspected nephrotic syndrome Multi-organ disease
Full blood count and film	Anaemia, infection, haemolysis
Coagulation	Septicaemia, disseminated intravascular coagulation (N.B. correct coagulopathy prior to kidney biopsy)

Figure 4.4 Laboratory investigation of acute renal failure

Test	Indication/abnormality
Blood cultures	Septicaemia Repeat if suspected endocarditis
Lactate dehydrogenase	Tissue infarction, haemolysis
Anti-neutrophil cytoplasmic antibody (ANCA)	Rapidly progressive glomerulonephritis (RPGN)
Anti-glomerular basement membrane (anti-GBM) antibody	RPGN
Antinuclear antibodies (ANA)	Systemic lupus erythematosus (SLE)
Complement components (C3, C4)	Decreased concentrations in SLE, endocarditis and cryoglobulinaemia
Cryoglobulins	Cryoglobulinaemia
Serum uric acid	Urate nephropathy
Serum protein electrophoresis	Myeloma
Anti-streptolysin O titre (ASOT)	Post-streptococcal glomerulonephritis
Virology	Hepatitis B & C, human immunodeficiency virus

Figure 4.4 cont. Laboratory investigation of acute renal failure

A kidney biopsy is reserved for cases of ARF where an ultrasound scan has excluded obstructed kidneys and the renal sizes are maintained. Small kidneys (< 9.0 cm) indicate long standing disease and kidney biopsy is unlikely to change management. Occasionally obstruction may exist in the setting of a non-dilated urinary tract, usually as a result of encasement from tumour. Alternative investigations in equivocal cases include CT scan and retrograde studies of the ureters and kidney collecting systems following direct visualisation of the bladder and selective cannulation of each ureteric orifice (Figure 4.5). The latter procedure is invasive and is performed by a specialist urologist.

Additional studies in acute renal failure	
Investigation	**Indication/abnormality**
Chest X-ray	Pulmonary oedema, pneumonia, effusions, pulmonary haemorrhage, granulomas, malignancy, bone lesions
Ultrasound scan of renal tract	Exclude dilated system Presence and size of two kidneys Small kidneys in advanced CKD Kidney stones
Computer assisted tomography (CT) scanning	Renal anatomy Kidney stones Malignancy Perfusion Aortic dissection
Renal angiography or magnetic resonance angiography	Critical renal artery stenosis Aortic dissection
Kidney biopsy (specialist renal unit only)	Unexplained ARF Suspected rapidly progressive glomerulo-nephritis
Cystoscopy and retrograde pyelography	Suspected obstruction

Figure 4.5 Additional studies in acute renal failure

Metabolic complications and management of ARF

Metabolic acidosis is the commonest acid-base disorder in patients with ARF. Reduced renal excretion of potassium and the effect of acidosis on the movement of potassium to the extracellular space may lead to a very high concentration of potassium in the plasma. Severe hyperkalaemia (serum potassium concentration > 6.5 mmol/L) is associated with life-threatening cardiac arrhythmias (Figure 4.6) and should be treated as outlined in Figure 4.7. The use of isotonic sodium bicarbonate can be considered as part of the crystalloid replacement fluid in patients with ARF. Dialysis is indicated in patients who do not improve despite attempts at correction. The options for RRT include intermittent haemodialysis, peritoneal dialysis and 'continuous' therapies (haemofiltration and haemodiafiltration). The

RRT modalities are discussed in detail in Chapter 7. The continuous modalities are particularly appropriate for the intensive care unit setting in cases of multi-organ failure. Indications for initiation of dialysis include refractory hyperkalaemia, pericarditis, pulmonary oedema not responding to diuretics and uraemic encephalopathy.

ECG abnormalities in hyperkalaemia

- Tented or peaked T waves

- Prolonged PR and QT intervals and widened QRS complexes

- Small or absent P waves

- Sine waves

- Ventricular fibrillation and asystole

Figure 4.6 ECG abnormalities in hyperkalaemia

Poisoning and ARF

Dialysis and haemoperfusion may be used in the treatment of drug overdose and poisoning in association with ARF. These procedures are rarely necessary and should only be considered after specialist advice from a poisons unit. Haemodialysis is suitable for low molecular weight, water soluble drugs that will diffuse rapidly across the dialysis membrane. Haemoperfusion involves the passage of blood through a cartridge packed with a sorbent, such as polymer-coated activated charcoal. The rationale is that the poison will be adsorbed to the charcoal and removed from the blood. Both procedures are more efficient at removing drugs confined to the vascular compartment compared to drugs that have a high volume of distribution. Haemodialysis is suitable for drugs with a low volume of distribution that are not protein bound and are water soluble. Examples include methanol and ethylene glycol (following ingestion of anti-freeze), lithium, aspirin, theophylline to a limited extent, and barbiturates. By contrast, tricyclic antidepressants and phenothiazines are highly protein bound and are not readily cleared by haemodialysis. Haemoperfusion is the preferred option for removing low molecular weight drugs with a low volume of distribution that are lipid soluble and protein bound. Examples of drugs and chemicals removed by haemoperfusion include theophylline, barbiturates and paraquat.

Treatment of hyperkalaemia

Serum potassium concentration > 6.5 mmol/L or ECG changes suggestive of hyperkalaemia

Immediate treatment

- 10 mL 10% calcium gluconate infusion over 10 minutes through a large bore venous cannula

- 50 mL 50% glucose intravenous infusion over 30 mins via a large bore venous cannula with 8-10 units of short-acting insulin with monitoring of glucose concentration (risk of hypoglycaemia following insulin)

- 500-1000 mL of isotonic sodium bicarbonate (1.26 or 1.4%) by intravenous infusion as part of crystalloid fluid replacement

Additional interventions

- Ion-exchange resins (e.g. calcium resonium) 15-30 g 8 hourly orally or by enema

- β_2-agonists

- Review drug list, removing nephrotoxic agents

- Repeat serum potassium measurements hourly until there is a sustained fall in concentration

- If potassium concentration is not falling, consider urgent transfer for dialysis or haemofiltration on the intensive care unit

Figure 4.7 Treatment of hyperkalaemia

Contrast nephropathy

Many procedures and tests that are undertaken within the hospital environment may contribute to the burden of ARF. In particular, diagnostic imaging using contrast-enhanced CT scanning and angiographic procedures account for the majority of cases of contrast-induced ARF. This is an important area since new contrast agents are being developed that are evidently safer in those patients that are at high risk of developing ARF when undergoing imaging. Radiocontrast media are iodinated and are either ionic or non-ionic. At the concentrations required for angiography or CT scanning, the various agents used have differing osmolalities. First generation agents were ionic monomers with a very high osmolality with respect to plasma (in the region of 1500-1800 mmol/kg). Second generation agents, such as iohexol are non-ionic monomers with a lower osmolality compared to first generation but still much higher than plasma (in the region of 600-850 mmol/kg). Recently, an iso-osmolal agent, iodixanol, has been introduced (290 mmol/kg), which may be less likely to cause ARF in high risk subjects.

Although minor increments of serum creatinine concentration are expected following adminitration of contrast, more marked decline in function is likely to occur in patients with one or more of the following risk factors:

- pre-existing kidney disease with GFR < 60 mL/min/1.73 m^2
- diabetic nephropathy
- hypovolaemia
- high dose of contrast agent

The pathogenesis of contrast mediated nephrotoxicity is not fully understood, but is thought to be a combination of renal vasoconstriction, regional hypoxia and production of reactive oxygen species causing direct tubular injury.

Patients undergoing percutaneous coronary interventions for coronary artery disease are particularly at risk. Approximately 25% of patients undergoing the procedure develop ARF, defined in this setting as a rise in serum creatinine concentration of 44 μmol/L (0.5 mg/dL) if the baseline creatinine is above 177 μmol/L (2.0 mg/dL). The use of iso-osmolar agents may lower the risk of ARF in high risk diabetic patients undergoing angiography. Preventative measures should be considered prior to administering a contrast load regardless of the contrast used. If possible, alternative investigations should be performed. However, in those patients that require radiocontrast, adequate hydration should be ensured using either normal saline or isotonic sodium bicarbonate. The antioxidant N-acetylcysteine is commonly used to prevent contrast nephropathy. There is no clear evidence of benefit, but it is well tolerated and safe. NSAIDs should be avoided in patients at risk of contrast nephropathy as they interfere with vasodilator prostaglandins, causing increased renal vasoconstriction.

Conclusion

ARF is common in patients admitted to hospital and in many cases is exacerbated by iatrogenic procedures and can be prevented. Clarification of the definition of ARF may enable comparisons to be made in future clinical trials and allow for early intervention in patients at high risk of ARF. Although the majority of cases of ARF fall into pre-renal causes and ATN, a standard approach to the investigation of ARF will help alert the medical team to the more unusual causes such as a rapidly progressive glomerulonephritis. The majority of patients can be managed on general wards; however, those patients with multi-organ failure require intensive care support and RRT. The clinical biochemistry laboratory provides invaluable support by identifying patients with ARF and enabling monitoring of biochemical derangement during the illness and during recovery of kidney function. The laboratory will also contribute to reaching the underlying diagnosis when kidney disease and systemic disease affecting the kidneys is suspected. The pathophysiology of ischaemic ATN has been described and to understand this requires knowledge of the basic principles of renal physiology including blood flow and tubular function. At present there are no effective therapeutic interventions over and above adequate fluid replacement in pre-renal ARF and ATN (Figure 4.8).

Summary of approach to a patient with acute renal failure

- Establish whether acute or acute on chronic renal failure

- Identify immediately whether pre-renal component and resuscitate with fluids

- Discontinue nephrotoxic drugs

- Treat metabolic complications

- Exclude urinary tract obstruction

- Investigate for parencyhmal disease

- Early discussion with local renal unit if not responding to immediate treatment

Figure 4.8 Summary of approach to a patient with acute renal failure

Further reading

Barrett BJ, Parfre, PS. Preventing nephropathy induced by contrast medium. N Engl J Med 2006; **354:** 379-86.

Bonventre JV, Weinberg JM. Recent advances in the pathophysiology of ischemic acute renal failure. J Am Soc Nephrol 2003; **14:** 2199-210.

Glynne P, Allen A and Pusey C (eds). Acute renal failure in practice. Imperial College Press, London UK. 2002 ISBN 1-86094-287-3.

Mehta RL, Chertow GM. Acute renal failure definitions and classification: time for change? J Am Soc Nephrol 2003; **14:** 2178-87.

Stevens PE, Tamimi NA, Al Hasani MK, Mikhail AI, Kearney E, Lapworth R *et al*. Non-specialist management of acute renal failure. Q J Med 2001; **94:** 533-40.

Van Biesen W, Vanholder R, Lamiere N. Defining acute renal failure: RIFLE and beyond. Clin J Am Soc Nephrol 2006; **1:** 1314-9

Chapter 5

Investigation and monitoring of specific kidney diseases

Diabetic nephropathy

Diabetes mellitus is a state of chronic hyperglycaemia sufficient to cause long-term damage to specific tissues, notably the retina, kidney, nerves, and arteries. It affects 176 million people worldwide and the prevalence is increasing rapidly. In the UK, 3% of the population have diabetes. Tissue lesions are common to both type 1 and type 2 diabetes. Diabetic nephropathy is a clinical diagnosis based on the finding of persistent proteinuria in a patient with diabetes. The earliest sign of nephropathy is the appearance of low level, but abnormal, albumin excretion; patients with a urinary albumin excretion rate between 30-300 mg/24 h (~3-30 mg/mmol creatinine) have microalbuminuria (see Chapter 3) and are said to have 'incipient nephropathy'. Without intervention, most patients with incipient nephropathy progress to overt diabetic nephropathy ('macroalbuminuria'), characterised by protein excretion exceeding 500 mg/24 h (equivalent to an albumin excretion rate of approximately 300 mg/24 h or > 30 mg/mmol creatinine). As albuminuria worsens and blood pressure increases, there is a relentless decline in GFR, albeit at a highly variable rate. ESRD develops in > 75% of patients with overt nephropathy over 20 years. However, intervention can affect the rate of decline. Diabetic nephropathy increases cardiovascular mortality and is the most common single cause of ESRD, accounting for approximately 40% of incident patients onto RRT programmes in the US compared with 20% in the UK. Among patients who require dialysis, those with diabetes have a 22% higher mortality at one year and a 15% higher mortality at five years than patients without diabetes.

Clinically, diabetic nephropathy develops slowly, but ultrastructural evidence of glomerular damage has been found in renal biopsies taken from type 1 diabetic patients within a few years of diagnosis. In type 1 diabetes, early macroscopic changes include kidney enlargement and pallor. With disease progression the kidneys become smaller. Type 2 diabetes is typified by variable kidney contraction due to associated ischaemia. On histological examination, glomerular changes include: diffuse mesangial sclerosis with matrix accumulation and irregularly thickened basement membranes, sclerotic, acellular mesangial nodules (so-called Kimmelstiel-Wilson lesions), hyaline fibrin cap lesions around peripheral capillary loops, capsular drop lesions located within Bowman's capsule and hyalinosis of arterioles (Plate 4).

Clinical progression is defined in terms of changes in urinary albumin excretion rate, decline in GFR and increase in blood pressure (Figure 5.1), although it should be noted that some patients with diabetes may show a decline in GFR in the absence of microalbuminuria. In type 1 diabetes, it is unusual to develop microalbuminuria within the first five years of diagnosis, but it can develop anytime thereafter, even after 40 years. The onset of type 2 diabetes is difficult to define and a higher proportion of patients are found to have microalbuminuria at diagnosis. Since microalbuminuria is the earliest sign of diabetic nephropathy and diabetic nephropathy can be ameliorated by treatment, routine screening of patients for microalbuminuria is recommended. This is discussed in Chapter 3.

Stages of diabetic nephropathy

Stage designation		Characteristics	Structural changes	GFR (mL/min/ 1.73 m^2)	Blood pressure (mm Hg)
I	Hyperfunction	Hyperfiltration	Glomerular hypertrophy	>150	Normal
II	Normoalbuminuria	Normal AER (<20 μg/min, <30 mg/24h)	Basement membrane thickening	150	Normal
III	Incipient diabetic nephropathy	Elevated AER (20-200 μg/min, (30-300 mg/24h)	AER correlates with structural damage and hypertrophy of remaining glomeruli	125	Increased
IV	Overt diabetic nephropathy	Clinical proteinuria (AER >200 μg/min, >300 mg/24 h)	Advanced structural damage	<100	Increased
V	Uraemia	ESRD	Glomerular closure	0-10	Increased

AER = albumin excretion rate, ESRD = end-stage renal disease, GFR = glomerular filtration rate.

Figure 5.1 Stages of diabetic nephropathy.

Pathophysiology of diabetic nephropathy
Diabetic nephropathy appears to be promoted by a variety of factors including hyperglycaemia, hypertension, hyperlipidaemia and proteinuria. However, these factors need to occur against a background of genetic susceptibility; only 30-40% of diabetic patients will develop nephropathy irrespective of glycaemic control.

Further evidence of genetic susceptibility has come from family studies and epidemiological studies, which have demonstrated ethnic differences in the prevalence of diabetic nephropathy. However, the disease is not described by a simple Mendelian inheritance model.

Hyperglycaemia is the common feature of the diabetic state and is almost certainly primarily responsible for the secondary complications of diabetes. Hyperglycaemic tissue damage probably arises via a series of mechanisms. A key step linking glucotoxicity to cellular dysfunction in diabetic nephropathy is the excess of extracellular matrix within the glomerulus and interstitium. The exposure of the kidney to hyperglycaemic conditions appears to induce transcription of the gene for TGF-β, which in turn upregulates the insulin-independent GLUT-1 transporter in mesangial cells. Glucose is transported into the cells through GLUT-1 and over-expression of GLUT-1 accelerates glucose-induced changes in the mesangial cells, including extracellular matrix accumulation.

Glomerular TGF-β mRNA is markedly increased in kidney biopsy specimens from patients with proven diabetic kidney disease. Blood and urine sampling across the renal vascular bed confirms net renal production of TGF-β in diabetic patients. Anti-TGF-β monoclonal antibodies can ameliorate the prosclerotic and hypertrophic effects of high ambient glucose concentrations in cultured renal cells and reverse established nephropathy in animal models. Activation of the renin-angiotensin-aldosterone system as a result of hypertension, a common feature of diabetes, may further exacerbate these changes through AII-stimulated TGF-β release. Treatment with ACE inhibitors lowers circulating TGF-β concentrations in patients with diabetic nephropathy. Advanced glycation end (AGE) products may further stimulate TGF-β production, both directly and through release of reactive oxygen species. AGEs may also have direct effects on matrix accumulation in addition to glomerular permeability effects via the podocyte AGE receptor. A further promoter of TGF-β, protein kinase C-β1 (PKC-β1) is a candidate gene for diabetic nephropathy. Haemodynamic dysfunction (systemic and glomerular hypertension and hyperfiltration) induces mechanical stretch and proteinuria via induction of vascular permeability factor mRNA; *in vitro* shear stress has also been shown to induce TGF-β production and GLUT-1 over-expression. However, there are conflicting reports as to whether hyperfiltration alone could cause glomerular changes in humans.

Treatment of diabetic nephropathy
Both the Diabetes Control and Complications Trial (DCCT) and the United Kingdom Prospective Diabetes Study (UKPDS) have shown that intensive diabetes therapy (strict glycaemic control) can significantly reduce the risk of development of nephropathy. Clinical guidelines for diabetes management, for

example those produced by NICE, set treatment targets defined in terms of glycated haemoglobin, with the aim of reducing the complication rate, including nephropathy. In addition, aggressive antihypertensive treatment can ameliorate the rate of fall in GFR and targets for blood pressure control are tighter for diabetic than for non-diabetic patients. The use of ACE inhibitors or ARBs appears to be particularly beneficial in this setting. These drugs appear to reduce albuminuria and the rate of decline in GFR to a greater extent than other antihypertensive agents for an equivalent reduction in blood pressure, presumably through intra-glomerular effects on capillary blood pressure and protein filtration. ACE inhibitors or ARBs may exacerbate hyperkalaemia in patients with advanced renal insufficiency, especially in the presence of renal artery stenosis. Dietary protein restriction, smoking cessation and reduction of LDL-cholesterol may have further beneficial effects on diabetic nephropathy.

Hypertension and the kidney

Blood pressure (BP), like other characteristics such as weight and height, shows intra-and inter-individual variation and will change at different times in an individual's life depending on genetic and environmental factors. In Western cultures, BP tends to rise with age and this was previously accepted as normal. The BP cut-off point that defines hypertension is arbitrary and based on the risk to the population being described. Using a cut-off point of 140/90 mmHg, the prevalence of hypertension in those aged 18-29 years is 4% and reaches 65% in those over 80 years. Population studies have confirmed that above certain levels of BP, there is an increased risk of cardiovascular disease and death. This effect is amplified if there are other risk factors such as diabetes, cigarette smoking and dyslipidaemia. In the Framingham Heart Study* heart failure developed six times as often in individuals classified as hypertensive (> 140/90 mmHg) compared with normotensive subjects. This study also found an impressive relationship between hypertension and risk of stroke and coronary heart disease (CHD). For example, a 5 mmHg lower diastolic BP and a 9 mm Hg lower systolic BP reduced the risk of stroke by 33% and CHD by 20%.

* The Framingham Heart Study commenced in 1948 and followed 5000 individuals from Framingham, Massachusetts, USA. It reports on outcome at regular intervals. Second and third generation cohorts have been recruited and risk factors for cardiovascular disease identified.

Major trials in hypertensive subjects have explored whether treating hypertension is beneficial in terms of mortality and cardiovascular morbidity. The epidemiological evidence suggests that the lower the BP, the greater the improvement in cardiovascular risk. For example, the Hypertension Optimal Treatment (HOT) Study conducted in 26 countries evaluated the relationship between three levels of target diastolic BP (< 80, < 85, or < 90 mmHg) and cardiovascular morbidity and mortality in hypertensive patients. Almost 20,000 patients aged between 50 and 80 years were studied. The lowest risk of major cardiovascular events occurred at a mean BP of 139/83 mmHg. There are a number of published national and international guidelines on the treatment of hypertension, although variability exists between their recommendations. The recently published Joint National Committee on Prevention, Detection, Evaluation and Treatment of High Blood Presssure (JNC VII) suggests that the risk of cardiovascular disease doubles for each increment of BP of 20/10 mmHg beginning at 115/75 mmHg. The report identifies 120/80 mmHg as normotension. All patients with hypertension (> 140/90 mmHg) should receive lifestyle change advice and antihypertensive medication if necessary.

The majority of hypertension is 'essential' hypertension. An underlying correctable medical cause can be identified in approximately 5% of patients: of these, half may have evidence of kidney disease. Kidney disease may include parenchymal diseases or specifically, a narrowing of a renal artery referred to as renal artery stenosis.

Hypertension and CKD
Hypertension and CKD are inevitably intertwined and in many circumstances it is difficult to identify whether the raised BP is causing kidney disease or *vice versa*. Hypertension is second only to diabetes as a primary diagnosis of ESRD for patients commencing dialysis in the US. In the 10 years to 2000, there was a 30% increase in hypertension as the primary cause of ESRD. The incidence is higher in the elderly and especially amongst the black American population. Although hypertension co-exists with CKD, there are situations where hypertension *per se* has caused CKD and may act as an accelerating force in the development of ESRD. Episodes of accelerated or 'malignant' hypertension can cause end-organ damage and, although usually effectively treated with antihypertensive drugs, may cause kidney failure. Patients with CKD and hypertension without a primary renal disease may have hypertensive nephropathy. Characteristic findings are seen on kidney biopsy and include vascular injury with vessel wall hyperplasia, glomerular scarring (sclerosis) and evidence of previous accelerated hypertension. Hypertension often develops as a consequence of CKD due to alterations in salt and water metabolism and activation of the sympathetic nervous system and renin-angiotensin system.

Treatment of hypertension to pre-defined target BP values is critical for prevention of progression to ESRD. Evidence from major clinical trials of BP lowering therapy, in patients with CKD and those in the general population without CKD, confirms that BP reduction is beneficial to much lower levels than previously thought. Some of this data has been described in Chapter 2. It is widely accepted that the majority of patients with CKD will require a combination of three to four antihypertensive drugs to reach these targets. The treatment regimen should include diuretics and agents to block the renin-angiotensin system. ACE inhibitors are more effective than other antihypertensive drugs in slowing the rate of progression of CKD, particularly if proteinuria is present. Short-term studies show that ARBs have effects on blood pressure and proteinuria that are similar to those of ACE inhibitors.

Renovascular disease
Selected patients may be referred to the nephrology clinic for evaluation of CKD and identification of underlying renovascular disease. There has been a significant increase in the identification of renal artery disease as a cause of ESRD, particularly in the elderly. Primary diseases of the renal arteries usually involve the origin of the renal arteries at the aorta (ostial lesions). Secondary disease with hypertension and chronic renal insufficiency with small-vessel and intrarenal disease is referred to as ischaemic nephropathy. There is a complex interplay between renal artery stenosis and ischaemic nephropathy. Atheromatous disease accounts for > 90% of renal artery stenosis. Atheromatous disease is progressive and may cause complete occlusion. The prevalence increases with age and is associated with particular clinical features (Figure 5.2). As a marker of established cardiovascular disease, ARAS is associated with a poor prognosis. Renal artery atheroma is found in up to 50% of post-mortems on elderly patients and up to 50% of patients undergoing angiography for coronary or peripheral vascular disease.

Patients who receive ACE inhibitors and ARBs may develop ARF and hyperkalaemia in the presence of severe bilateral renal artery stenosis or severe disease to a single functioning kidney, since in these settings AII-dependent mechanisms are maintaining kidney function. Kidney function should be carefully monitored following the introduction of these drugs. A 10-15% reduction in GFR should be considered a normal physiological response to renin-angiotensin system blockade and a small increment in plasma creatinine concentration consistent with this should be tolerated, provided that it is not progressive. Marked deterioration in kidney function following introduction of these agents should raise the suspicion of renovascular disease. The diagnosis is important to make, since radiological deployment of intraluminal stents is possible and surgical repair can be performed to improve patency of the vessel. To place this in context, a correctable

ARAS lesion is found in fewer than 1% of all hypertensive patients. Investigation, therefore, has to be targeted to high risk groups.

Renal artery stenosis in younger patients is characteristically due to fibromuscular dysplasia. The medial part of the artery is most commonly affected and presents radiologically as alternate bands of narrowing and dilatation, giving rise to a 'string of beads' appearance. If the diagnosis is made, hypertension can be cured in at least 50% of cases following balloon angioplasty to the artery.

Clinical features associated with renal artery stenosis
New hypertension in young person < 30 y or older person > 60 y
Smoker
Diabetes
Associated macrovascular disease
Refractory hypertension
Renal asymmetry on ultrasound scan
Renal or other vascular bruit
Renal failure following blockade of renin-angiotensin system

Figure 5.2 Clinical features associated with renal artery stenosis.

Investigation of hypertension

It is recommended that all patients with hypertension should have some baseline tests performed. Primary investigations are performed to aid diagnosis of a specific cause, but equally importantly to detect hypertensive end-organ damage. Urinalysis is the simplest and often most revealing basic investigation of hypertension. Haematuria and proteinuria may identify patients with underlying kidney disease and hypertensive nephrosclerosis. In cases of hypertension where proteinuria is present, the risk of death is doubled for a given level of BP. Plasma electrolyte and creatinine concentrations should be measured to detect hypokalaemia (suggestive of hyperaldosteronism, including Conn's syndrome) and to assess kidney function. A lipid profile is also mandatory to assess overall cardiovascular risk. Severe hypertension is often associated with hyper-reninaemia, giving rise to secondary hyperaldosteronism characterised by a hypokalaemic metabolic alkalosis. Physiological stimulation of renin release occurs in the presence of hypotension, decreased sodium intake and dehydration.

Nearly all diuretics and antihypertensive agents affect renin release. When evaluating the renin-angiotensin system these agents should be tapered and discontinued two weeks before sampling (longer for spironolactone), although this can prove difficult in clinical practice.

Diagnosis of renal artery stenosis requires a high index of suspicion and is guided by radiological examination of the renal arterial anatomy (Figure 5.3). The gold standard is selective renal angiography, although the introduction of magnetic resonance angiography accurately diagnoses significant (> 50-70%) stenosis in the majority of cases and is noninvasive.

Investigation of suspected renal artery stenosis	
Test	**Observation**
Renal ultrasound	Ensure kidneys > 8 cm and check for symmetry. ARAS suspected if renal asymmetry.
Radionucleotide scintigraphy: DMSA (dimercaptosuccinic acid)	Differential function between each kidney can be identified
Captopril renogram	Can be useful in hypertensive patients with normal kidney function. ACE inhibitor (captopril) is administered and if the transit time of the radiotracer within the kidney increases significantly this suggests renal artery stenosis. The test is less useful in patients with renal impairment and in bilateral disease.
Spiral CT scanning	Where available, can give detailed images of arterial tree. In patients with CKD there is a risk of contrast nephropathy.
MRI with renal angiography	Safe and noninvasive. Surface-rendering software allows striking images of arterial anatomy to be produced.
Selective renal artery angiography	Gold standard for diagnosis. Patients can be recalled for balloon angioplasty and intraluminal stent deployment.

Figure 5.3 Investigation of suspected renal artery stenosis (ARAS)

Glomerular diseases

Glomerular disease is suggested clinically by the finding of blood and protein in the urine. Proteinuria of more than 1 g/24 hours (~100 mg/mmoL creatinine), in the absence of an overflow type proteinuria such as myoglobinuria or light chain related disease, is invariably glomerular in origin. Although a detailed discussion of each glomerular disease is beyond the scope of this book, the most important diseases will be discussed to illustrate the spectrum of disease. The incidence of ESRD in the Western world has increased dramatically over recent years. During this time there has been no change in the incidence of primary glomerular diseases causing ESRD in the US. Proven glomerulonephritis (GN) accounts for 10% of new cases of ESRD in the UK.

Primary glomerular diseases

GN can be primary (affecting only the kidneys) or secondary, in which the kidneys are involved as part of a systemic process. The histopathological classification of GN may appear slightly cumbersome, but is readily simplified by consideration of the glomerular structures and cells that may be involved and the presence or absence of immune complexes (Figure 5.4). There are only three cell types involved (endothelial, epithelial and mesangial), as well as the glomerular basement membrane (GBM). The glomerular cells and GBM have a limited range of responses to injury, i.e. proliferation, scarring (sclerosis) and GBM thickening. The term 'focal' is used if fewer than half of the glomeruli are involved in the disease process, as seen on light microscopy (LM). Diffuse GN refers to more widespread involvement of the glomeruli when viewed by LM. Immune deposits identified following immunofluorescence or immunoperoxidase (IM) staining, do not define whether a disease is focal or diffuse.

IgA nephropathy is an example of a focal GN, with focal mesangial cell proliferation demonstrated by LM. There is however, diffuse and global deposition of the immunoglobulin, IgA (Plate 5). It is the most common type of GN worldwide and has a particularly high prevalence around the Pacific rim. The disease tends to be slowly progressive depending, as with most kidney diseases, on the degree of proteinuria and kidney function at diagnosis and degree of interstitial fibrosis on biopsy. Up to 50% of patients exhibit elevated concentrations of serum IgA, although diagnosis depends on kidney biopsy findings. Clinical presentation varies considerably, from asymptomatic microscopic haematuria to macroscopic haematuria; proteinuria including nephrotic syndrome and kidney failure. Episodic macroscopic haematuria is seen in some patients at the same time as an upper respiratory tract infection. IgA nephropathy may also present with established proteinuria, renal impairment and hypertension. The variation in clinical and histological features leads to difficulties in reaching conclusions regarding treatment protocols that have been tested in clinical trials. Biopsy findings are pathognomonic with mesangial deposition of polymeric IgA (pIgA). In most cases there is associated deposition of IgG and IgM. Complement factors, such as C3, are also deposited in the same distribution as IgA. The mesangial matrix accumulates as disease progresses. Crescents may be seen during episodes of macroscopic haematuria. Tubulointerstitial changes are consistent with other forms of kidney disease, reflecting a common pathway of fibrosis. Electron microscopy (EM) confirms electron-dense deposits within the mesangium.

Overview of primary glomerular diseases

Disease	Histological findings	Clinical spectrum	Treatment	Prognosis
IgA nephropathy	Focal mesangial cell proliferation on LM. IgA deposited within mesangial cells on IM.	Variable: incidental finding; episodes of macroscopic haematuria; proteinuria; declining GFR. There is a male preponderence and the peak incidence occurs in the second and third decades of life. May be associated with systemic vasculitis in HSP.	Generic treatment targeting BP and RAAS blockade. Selected cases receive corticosteroids and cytotoxic drugs.	Variable, but 30-40% progress to ESRD over 20 years.
Minimal change nephropathy	Little evidence of cellular involvement on LM. Podocyte foot process effacement demonstrated on EM. No immune deposits.	Most common cause of nephrotic syndrome in children. Usually idiopathic. Relapsing and remitting course.	Oral corticosteroids and cytotoxic drugs.	Does not cause ESRD. Significant side effects of immunosuppressant drugs.
FSGS	Glomerular scarring and non-specific trapping of immune complexes in scarred areas.	Common cause of nephrotic syndrome in adults. Congenital forms described. Secondary causes include collapsing variety seen in HIVAN.	Idiopathic disease requires corticosteroids and cytotoxic drugs in selected cases.	Nephrotic syndrome commonly refractory to treatment. 30-40% develop ESRD at 10 years.

Figure 5.4 Overview of primary glomerular diseases

Disease	Histological findings	Clinical spectrum	Treatment	Prognosis
Membranous nephropathy	Thickened GBM with immune deposits in sub-epithelial GBM. Classically 'spikes' are seen along the GBM and represent new GBM squeezed between deposits.	Common cause of nephrotic syndrome. Secondary cause in 20% of cases.	Treat underlying condition. If idiopathic treat generically and if progressive, add immuno-suppressive drug.	Variable outcome; 'rule of thirds' (see text).
MCGN (types I, II & III)	Mixed mesangial cell proliferation with GBM thickening. Immune complexes may be seen (types I & III).	May be idiopathic or associated with persistent infections (SBE, hepatitis B, C & HIV, malaria) and systemic diseases (SLE and cryoglobulinaemia, malignancy and lymphoma). A rare association of MCGN with persistent activation of the alternate complement pathway by a circulating C3 nephritic factor and partial lipodystrophy is recognised.	Treat underlying disease. Cortico-steroids and cytotoxic drugs (limited controlled data).	Depends on cause. Idiopathic MCGN has a variable course.

BP, blood pressure; EM, electron microscopy; ESRD, end-stage renal disease; FSGS, focal segmental glomerulosclerosis; GBM, glomerular basement membrane; HIV, human immunodeficiency virus; HIVAN, human immunodeficiency virus associated nephropathy; HSP, Henoch-Schonlein purpura; IM, immunofluo-rescence or immunoperoxidase microscopy; MCGN, mesangiocapillary glomerulonephritis; RAAS, renin-angiotensin-aldosterone system; SBE, subacute bacterial endocarditis; SLE, systemic lupus erythematosus.

Figure 5.4 cont. Overview of glomerular diseases

No treatment is available that specifically reduces mesangial deposition of IgA and available options are limited to modifying downstream immune and inflam-matory events that may lead to scarring. Treatment options include tonsillectomy for patients with macroscopic haematuria associated with respiratory infections or no treatment in those with isolated microscopic haematuria or low level proteinuria (< 1 g/24 h (~100 mg/mmol creatinine). In progressive disease all patients are treated in a similar generic fashion as for most kidney diseases. This includes reducing BP to < 125/75 mmHg and comprehensive renin-angiotensin-aldosterone system (RAAS) blockade to minimise proteinuria. An assessment of the impact of immunosuppressive therapies is compromised by the heterogeneity of the disease and the limited duration of randomised controlled studies with sufficient numbers to draw a conclusion. Nevertheless, a large Italian study with greater than 10 years of follow-up data demonstrates benefit from oral cortico-steroids in high doses for six months; there was a significant reduction in protein-uria and progression to ESRD in the treated patients. However, the cohort studies were not typically treated to the above defined generic guidelines for treatment of glomerular disease. In most UK practice, corticosteroids are generally reserved for patients with progressive disease despite optimal BP and maximum RAAS blockade. Corticosteroids are used to treat nephrotic syndrome that may occur in IgA nephropathy. Some evidence exists for the efficacy of the cytotoxic drug cyclophosphamide, followed by azathioprine in conjunction with high-dose pred-nisolone, in patients with IgA nephropathy that are at very high risk for progres-sion to ESRD. This is an unusual clinical scenario and therefore cyclophos-phamide is typically reserved for patients with crescentic IgA with rapidly progressive kidney failure. In summary, treatment of IgA nephropathy is prima-rily generic with BP reduction and use of ACE inhibitors and ARBs alone or in combination. Selected cases may be considered for immunosuppressive therapy.

NEPHROTIC SYNDROME
Nephrotic syndrome is defined as heavy proteinuria (> 3 g/24 h, ~300 mg/mmol creatinine), reduced serum albumin concentration and oedema. In comparison to nephritic syndrome, nephrotic patients may exhibit an otherwise bland urinary sediment with little haematuria. Nephrotic syndrome can occur at any age. Although the underlying kidney disease tends to vary with age, in all cases the lesion is within the glomerulus and is associated with damage to the specialised visceral epithelial cells, the podocytes (Chapter 1). Podocytes are characterised by large cell bodies and numerous foot processes. Foot processes are divided into primary and secondary, and the secondary processes interdigitate between adja-cent cells and are anchored to the GBM via integrin molecules and dystroglycans. The gap between interdigitating foot processes is called the slit diaphragm and forms the final barrier to filtration. Following the discovery of a number of genes and podocyte proteins that comprise the slit diaphragm, the pathophysiology of glomerular proteinuria is beginning to be elucidated (Figure 5.5).

Component molecules of the podocyte slit diaphragm

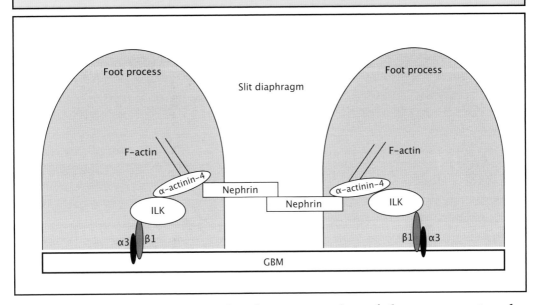

Figure 5.5 Schematic cross-sectional representation of the component molecules of the podocyte slit diaphragm and their interaction with the glomerular basement membrane (GBM) and foot processes. Nephrin was the first protein to be identified as crucial to maintaining the glomerular barrier to filtration following genetic studies of individuals with congenital nephrotic syndrome in Finland. Nephrin is a large transmembrane protein and a physical interaction has been described with proteins connecting to the GBM. These proteins include integrin ($\alpha 3$ and $\beta 1$) molecules, linked to the foot process cytoskeleton via integrin-linked kinase (ILK). Disruption to these molecules induces podocyte foot process effacement and heavy proteinuria. (Reproduced with permission from Chunsun D *et al.*, Essential role of integrin-linked kinase in podocyte biology: bridging the integrin and slit diaphragm signalling. J Am Soc Nephrol 2006; **17**: 2164-2175).

The most common causes of nephrotic syndrome are minimal change disease, focal segmental glomerulosclerosis (FSGS) and membranous nephropathy. Secondary causes are discussed separately and include diabetic nephropathy, AL-amyloid and SLE. Diagnosis can only be made on kidney biopsy, which is generally undertaken in all adult patients presenting with nephrotic syndrome. Nephrotic syndrome is associated with significant morbidity regardless of cause and patients with the condition have increased cardiovascular disease due to marked hyperlipidaemia, increased infection and risk of thromboembolic disease.

Between 10-40% of patients with nephrotic syndrome develop evidence of arterial and venous thromboemboli, particularly deep vein and renal vein thrombosis (DVT and RVT). RVT appears to be most common in nephrotic syndrome due to membranous nephropathy and mesangiocapillary GN (MCGN). RVT may be unilateral or bilateral and may extend into the inferior vena cava. However, most cases of RVT have an insidious onset and produce no symptoms. Infrequently, patients develop acute RVT and present with signs of renal infarction, including flank pain, microscopic or gross haematuria. In addition, ARF may supervene in cases of nephrotic syndrome (Figure 5.6) and prolonged proteinuria with a poor response to treatment may lead to ESRD.

Causes of acute renal failure in nephrotic syndrome
Acute tubular necrosis usually in minimal change disease and patients > 50 years of age
Minimal change disease with acute interstitial nephritis induced by NSAIDs
Tubular injury in collapsing focal segmental glomerulosclerosis: idiopathic or associated with HIV infection
Cresentic glomerulonephritis superimposed on membranous nephropathy

Figure 5.6 Causes of acute renal failure in nephrotic syndrome

The management of nephrotic syndrome depends upon the underlying glomerular lesion although general principles apply in all cases (Figure 5.7). Specific treatment targeted at inducing remission from proteinuria usually requires a combination of immunosuppressive drugs, including corticosteroids, and cytotoxic drugs.

Minimal change disease
Minimal change disease (MCD) is the most common cause of nephrotic syndrome in children and young adults. The incidence of MCD is estimated at 1-5 cases per 100,000 children per year. It typically presents with severe oedema and urine testing confirms heavy proteinuria. Kidney function is normal with little evidence of a reduced GFR. MCD does not progress to ESRD except in some cases of severe refractory disease that may be complicated by FSGS. Nephrotic syndrome in a non-infant child is assumed to be caused by MCD and a kidney biopsy is not generally performed. ARF can occur as a complication of nephrotic syndrome (Figure 5.6).

Management of nephrotic syndrome

Low sodium diet

Protein intake of 1.0 g/kg/day

Fluid management: usually includes loop diuretics (furosemide and bumetanide)

Thromboembolism prophylaxis: formal anticoagulation in high risk patients (serum albumin < 20 g/L or nephrotic syndrome due to membranous nephropathy or mesangiocapillary GN)

Vigilance for infections

Treatment of hyperlipidaemia with HMG-CoA-reductase inhibitors (statins)

Treatment of hypertension, primarily with RAAS blockade

Supportive treatment of ARF

Education and psychological support for patients and relatives

Figure 5.7 Management of nephrotic syndrome

A trial of treatment with corticosteroids characterises the steroid-responsiveness of the condition. Minimal change disease is typically steroid sensitive and may undergo a relapsing and remitting course. The most important prognostic indicator in nephrotic syndrome is steroid-responsiveness. In the majority of cases of MCD in children remission occurs within two weeks. Adults take slightly longer although the majority will be in remission within 4-6 weeks. Following disappearance of proteinuria, or one week after remission is induced, the corticosteroid dose can be reduced and tapered slowly. An attempt to withdraw treatment may be made after eight weeks. Longer duration of corticosteroid therapy significantly reduces the risk of relapse and many centres will treat for a minimum of 12 weeks, particularly with a first episode of steroid-responsive nephrotic syndrome. Around 60% of steroid-responsive patients experience multiple relapses. In addition to the comorbidity associated with nephrotic syndrome, the burden of long-term exposure to corticosteroids and cytotoxic drugs has to be considered. Cyclophosphamide, azathioprine and ciclosporin are reserved for refractory cases and can be used as corticosteroid-sparing agents with the aim of reducing relapse rates. Treatment with cyclophosphamide is limited to 8-12 weeks to reduce risk of gonadal toxicity. The cumulative dose threshold after which this risk increases significantly, is 200 mg/kg in children.

The histological lesion is by definition 'minimal' when viewed on light microscopy. However, electron microscopy confirms disruption to the epithelial surface of the glomerular capillary. Podocyte foot processes are detached (effaced) from the GBM, effectively removing the slit diaphragm and therefore the final barrier to filtration (Plate 6). The glomerular architecture is restored following prompt treatment with high dose corticosteroids. In MCD, the onset of nephrotic syndrome is often preceded by an infection or allergic reaction and it has been proposed that nephrotic syndrome may be the result of an exaggerated response to normal physiological and immune mechanisms that increase proteinuria during infection. MCD does occur in adults presenting with nephrotic syndrome. MCD occasionally complicates NSAID ingestion and secondary MCD has been described in patients with malignancy (particularly Hodgkin's lymphoma).

FOCAL SEGMENTAL GLOMERULOSCLEROSIS

FSGS (Plate 7) is the most important cause of the nephrotic syndrome in adults and remains a frequent cause in children and adolescents, particularly in the US, Brazil, and many other countries. A survey of renal biopsies performed from 1995 to 1997 for idiopathic nephrotic syndrome in adults in the US found that FSGS was the most common cause, accounting for 35% of all cases and > 50% among blacks. The relative roles of genetic and socioeconomic factors in explaining the increased susceptibility of blacks to FSGS are uncertain. Genetic studies in children with familial nephrotic syndrome characterised by FSGS have identified mutations in genes that encode important podocyte proteins. Nephrin was the first slit diaphragm protein identified and mutations in this transmembrane protein cause congenital (Finnish-type) nephrotic syndrome occurring with a frequency of 1/8200 live births in Finland. Among children with inherited nephrotic syndrome, mutations have been described in genes encoding other podocyte proteins (podocin, α-actinin 4, CD2-AP), all of which are crucial to the interaction of the slit diaphragm with the podocyte cytoskeleton (Figure 5.5). In young children with steroid-resistant nephrotic syndrome, genetic studies should be performed to identify mutations in genes coding for podocyte-specific proteins. Recently, podocin mutations have been observed to be present at high frequency among patients with sporadic forms of FSGS.

Compelling evidence suggests that a soluble permeability factor may be the cause of nephrotic syndrome in FSGS. This includes experience in kidney transplantation whereby FSGS may recur within hours of transplantation of a normal kidney into a patient reaching ESRD as a result of FSGS. The nature of the permeability factor remains unknown, but can be removed by immunoadsorption to protein A and plasma exchange prior to transplantation.

Although primary or idiopathic FSGS typically presents with an acute onset of nephrotic syndrome, secondary FSGS can occur and usually presents insidiously with non-nephrotic range proteinuria and reduction in GFR. Several disease processes lead to the description of FSGS on kidney biopsy and are shown in Figure 5.8.

Causes of secondary FSGS

Glomerular hypertrophy/hyperfiltration

     unilateral renal agenesis

     massive obesity

Scarring due to previous injury

     focal proliferative GN

     vasculitis

     systemic lupus erythematosus

Toxins (e.g. pamidronate)

Human immunodeficiency virus associated nephropathy (HIVAN)

Heroin nephropathy

Figure 5.8 Secondary causes of focal sclerosing glomerulosclerosis

Proteinuria in secondary FSGS, as in primary FSGS, reflects epithelial injury, although the mechanism is different. Following nephron loss, the remaining glomeruli undergo hypertrophy. Since podocytes are rarely able to replicate there is a decreased density of available foot processes to cover the enlarged glomerular surface. Focal areas of denudation from the glomerular basement membrane ensue, leading to proteinuria. The electron microscopic findings may also differ in primary and secondary FSGS. Primary FSGS is associated with diffuse foot process fusion, whereas in secondary FSGS, foot process fusion tends to be localised to sclerotic areas. Despite this, it is often very difficult to define on biopsy whether a primary or secondary process is occurring and the clinical features are paramount. This is important, since corticosteroids and other immunosuppressant drugs are not recommended for secondary or congenital forms of FSGS. It has long been considered that nephrotic syndrome complicating primary FSGS is largely corticosteroid-resistant with complete remission occurring in only 15-20% of adult cases. However, longer courses of steroids are now employed and corticosteroid resistance is not declared until at least six months of high dose treatment. Slow tapering of corticosteroid dose can occur once remission is established. The glomerular tip lesion variant of primary FSGS has been reported to have a more favourable response to corticosteroids, with complete or partial remission in 75% of cases.

MEMBRANOUS NEPHROPATHY

The term membranous nephropathy reflects the primary histological change noted on light microscopy (Plate 8): basement membrane thickening with little or no cellular proliferation or infiltration. Electron microscopy reveals electron-dense deposits across the GBM, particularly in the subepithelial space (Plate 9). The immune nature of these deposits is confirmed by immunohistochemistry with immunoglobulins and complement components readily demonstrated. Idiopathic membranous nephropathy is a common cause of nephrotic syndrome, accounting for approximately 30% of adult cases. The clinical progression is variable and is classically described as follows ('rule of thirds'):

- a third of patients undergo spontaneous remission of proteinuria and recovery of kidney function,
- a third of patients have non-progressive disease but evidence of ongoing proteinuria,
- a third of patients continue to exhibit nephrotic syndrome and are at high risk of progressive kidney failure.

The clinical course is therefore difficult to predict at the onset of the disease although 40% of patients develop ESRD after 10 years. Patients are generally observed for six months to assess the likely natural history of the condition and treated generically. A course of immunosuppressive drugs is indicated in progressive cases or those that have evidence of nephrotic syndrome for at least six months. Typical immunosuppressive schedules include high dose corticosteroids, calcineurin inhibitors such as ciclosporin, and cytotoxic drugs (chlorambucil and cyclophosphamide).

Secondary causes of membranous nephropathy are associated with a wide spectrum of diseases (see Figure 5.9). In comparison to idiopathic disease, the clinical outcome depends on the underlying disease process with subtle features on kidney biopsy suggesting a secondary process. These features include the concurrent presence of mesangial and subendothelial deposits in lupus nephritis, hepatitis B virus-induced disease and gold or penicillamine toxicity. In addition, the membranous variant of lupus nephritis is characterised by demonstration of IgG, C3 and C1q, and other immunoglobulins (referred to as a 'full house'). Underlying malignancy has been thought to be responsible for up to 5 to 10% of cases of membranous nephropathy in adults, the risk being highest in patients > 60 years of age. A solid tumour (such as carcinoma of the lung or colon) is most often involved and is usually clinically obvious. In the majority of cases the clinical features are those of the underlying disease.

Secondary causes of membranous nephropathy
Systemic lupus erythematosus
Hepatitis B
Falciparum malaria
Malignancy
Drugs (gold, penicillamine, captopril)

Figure 5.9 Secondary causes of membranous nephropathy

Systemic diseases causing glomerular disease

In all patients with glomerular disease it is important to consider whether an underlying systemic condition is present (Figure 5.10). There is often no clear distinction between primary and secondary glomerular diseases. As discussed above, both FSGS and membranous nephropathy may have secondary causes.

RAPIDLY PROGRESSIVE GLOMERULONEPHRITIS (RPGN)

RPGN is a heterogeneous group of disorders characterised by a fulminant clinical course that leads to kidney failure in only weeks or months. These syndromes are often characterised by focal necrotising GN and extracapillary crescent formation (crescentic glomerulonephritis, Plates 10 and 11) within the parietal layer of Bowman's capsules. Proliferating parietal epithelial cells and macrophages eventually compress the glomeruli and obstruct the proximal convoluted tubules, thus severely compromising nephron function. The proliferation of epithelial cells and macrophages occurs in response to fibrinogen and fibrin polymers present in Bowman's space. This is a non-specific reaction to severe glomerular injury attended by leakage of fibrinogen, activated enzymes and macrophages out of the capillaries into Bowman's space.

Overview of secondary glomerular diseases

Disease	Histological findings	Clinical spectrum	Treatment	Prognosis
RPGN	Capillary necrosis and parietal epithelial cell proliferation within Bowman's capsule with crescent formation. Vasculitis of extra-glomerular blood vessels may be seen. Lack of immune reactants ('pauci-immune'). In contrast, anti-GBM disease characterised by 100% crescents and linear GBM staining in IM.	May present as renal-limited small vessel vasculitis, or as part of a systemic vasculitis often associated with ANCA. Renal failure occurs over days and weeks if untreated. May be associated with pulmonary haemorrhage in life threatening cases.	Treatment with corticosteroids, cytotoxic drugs and plasma exchange.	Life-long follow-up. Prognosis improved from 90% mortality at 1 year to 20-30% with modern management. Patients with dialysis-dependent renal failure have less favourable outcome.
Diabetic nephropathy	Mesangial matrix expansion and thickening of GBM. Negative IM. Advanced cases of glomerular nodular sclerosis (K-W nodules).	Microalbuminuria to nephrotic syndrome and kidney failure.	See text	Commonest cause of ESRD in USA and most of Western Europe.
Dysproteinaemias	Amorphous acellular deposits within glomerulus and blood vessels stain positive with Congo Red. Light chain deposition disease may resemble nodular sclerosis lesions seen in diabetic nephropathy.	Primary AL-amyloid associated with nephrotic syndrome and kidney failure. Underlying plasma cell dyscrasia with increased production of monoclonal free light chains.	Common cause of nephrotic syndrome in the older person. Chemotherapy to reduce production of free monoclonal light chains.	Poor prognosis.

Figure 5.10 Overview of secondary glomerular diseases

Plates

The authors are extremely grateful to Dr Michael Lapsley, FRCPath for providing the following plates.

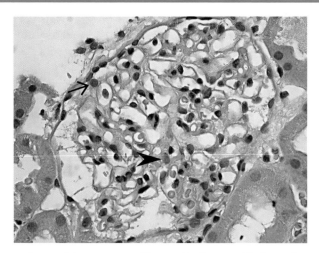

1. Normal glomerulus with surrounding tubules on light microscopy

The mesangium contains only a small amount of matrix and fewer than three mesangial nuclei (arrowhead) are visible per tuft. The capillary loops are open and thin and endothelial nuclei are infrequently visible. Podocyte nuclei (arrow) and cytoplasm can be seen within the urinary space. Erythrocytes can clearly be seen within the capillary loops. (Haematoxylin and eosin stain; objective x 60 magnification).

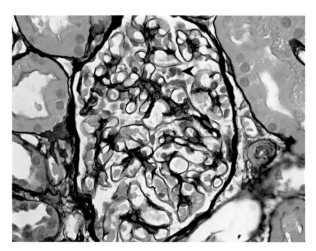

2. Normal glomerulus seen on light microscopy

The silver stain outlines the capillary loops by staining the basement membrane. Occasional endothelial nuclei are visible within the loops and podocytes (arrow head) can be located within the urinary space. The basement membrane is thin and even in texture. The mesangial cells are inconspicuous and each tuft contains one or two nuclei. (Combined silver/haematoxylin and eosin stain; objective x 60 magnification).

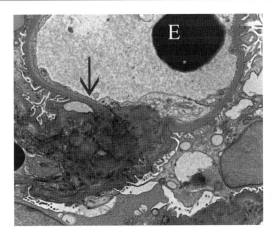

3. Normal glomerulus seen on electron microscopy

A capillary loop containing an erythrocyte (E) and lined by thin fenestrated endothelium (arrow). The endothelial nucleus does not happen to have been included in this section. The mesangium towards the bottom contains matrix and organelles. The three layers of the basement membrane can be seen, and then the podocyte foot process and, further away, the associated nuclei. The foot processes can most clearly be seen attached to the epithelial surface of the basement membrane at one to three o'clock.

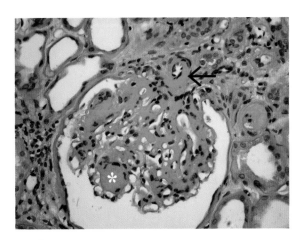

4. Diabetic nephropathy

This glomerulus shows expansion of the mesangium by amorphous eosinophilic material both diffusely and forming Kimmelstiel-Wilson nodules (*). Some capillary loops appear relatively normal while others show thickening of the basement membrane. At the hilum (arrow) a capillary with hyalinisation of the wall is present. The adjacent interstitium is inflamed with ischaemic damage to the tubules – this is commonly seen but is not specific to diabetic nephropathy. (Periodic acid-Schiff stain; objective x 60 magnification).

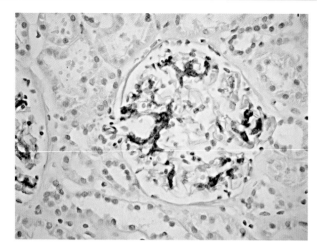

5. IgA nephropathy as seen following immunoperoxidase staining
Immunocytochemical (immunoperoxidase) staining of a glomerulus for IgA. The strong granular staining is confined to the mesangium. The capillary loops, which can be seen on the faint counter stain, are normal. IgA nephropathy typically shows mesangial proliferation on light microscopy (not shown), a non-specific finding. (Objective x 40 magnification).

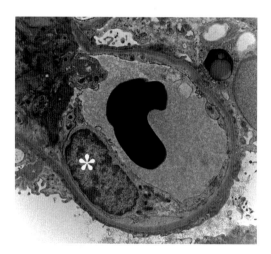

6. Foot process effacement in a patient with nephrotic syndrome
This shows a capillary loop containing a red cell and with an endothelial nucleus (*) visible. On the epithelial side of the basement membrane there is complete foot process effcaement with the podocyte cytoplasm adherent to the basement membrane in a continuous layer (compare with normal foot processes in plate 3). No deposits are present in this case of minimal change nephrotic syndrome.

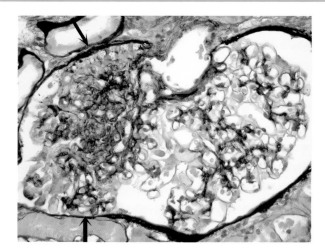

7. Focal segmental glomerulosclerosis (FSGS)

The right hand side of this glomerulus is relatively normal, but the tuft on the left shows sclerosis indicating the segmental nature of the lesion. There is increased staining density of the mesangium and loss of capillary lumina. The whole glomerulus is enlarged and is variably adherent to the Bowman's capsule (arrows). Although not shown, not all glomeruli are affected (i.e. the disease is focal). (Combined silver/haematoxylin and eosin stain; objective x 60 magnification).

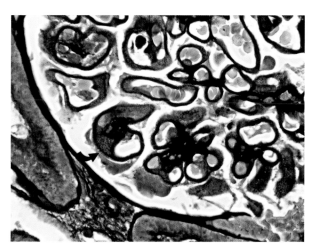

8. Membranous nephropathy as seen on light microscopy

Combined silver/haematoxylin and eosin stain showing basement membrane abnormalities. Small projections ('spikes', arrow) extend outwards towards the epithelial cells. These cause the glomerular basement membrane to have a mottled appearance where they are seen en-face ('bubbling artefact'). They represent sub-epithelial immune-complex deposition. (Combined silver/haematoxylin and eosin stain; objective x 100 magnification).

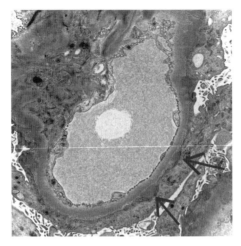

9. Membranous nephropathy as seen on electron microscopy
A capillary loop with the mesangium towards the upper left. On the epithelial side of the basement membrane there are numerous electron-dense deposits (arrows). The overlying podocyte foot processes are effaced and the podocyte epithelium is directly adherent to the basement membrane and the deposit. As the disease progresses the deposits will become surrounded by, and incorporated in, newly formed basement membrane material. It is the newly formed basement membrane that causes the spike appearance and not the electron-dense deposits.

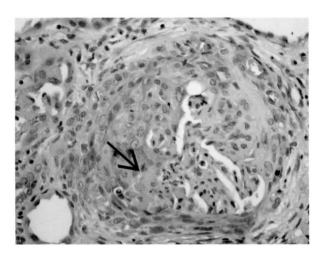

10. Small vessel vasculitis and crescent formation
The glomerular tuft is collapsed and inconspicuous with most of the Bowman's space being occupied by proliferating epithelial cells. Areas of necrosis (arrow) are present. This is crescentic glomerulonephritis and has similar appearances in pauci-immune vasculitis type glomerulonephritis and antiglomerular basement membrane disease. (Haematoxylin and eosin stain; objective x 40 magnification).

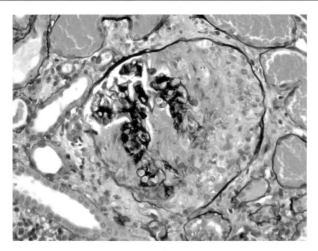

11. Small vessel vasculitis and crescent formation

The collapsed glomerular tuft is outlined by the silver stain while the majority of the Bowman's space is taken up with proliferating cellular crescent. Note the striking intratubular bleeding. (Combined silver/haematoxylin and eosin stain; objective x 60 magnification).

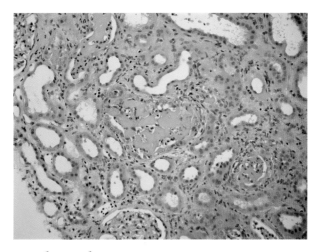

12. Myeloma cast nephropathy

The central tubule is distended by a pink staining fractured cast together with inflammatory cells. Two other tubules similarly affected can also be seen. The tubular epithelial cells are damaged and this is beginning to evoke a cellular response. Light chain restriction (i.e kappa or lambda) can often be demonstrated by immunocytochemistry within the casts. (Haematoxylin and eosin stain; objective x 20 magnification).

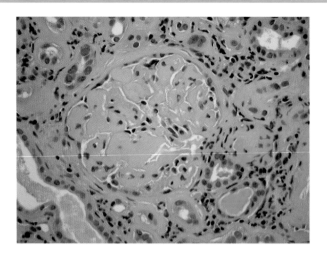

13. Amyloid

This glomerulus shows mesangial deposition of eosinophilic material, which appears dense and irregular, with loss of mesangial cellularity. The adjacent tubules are atrophic. Amyloid fibrils demonstrate apple-green birefringence when viewed under polarised light after staining with Congo red (not shown) and have a characteristic ultrastructure. (Haematoxylin and eosin stain; objective x 40 magnification).

Disease	Histological findings	Clinical spectrum	Treatment	Prognosis
Thrombotic microangiopathies	Microvascular thrombosis	Accelerated hypertension HUS/TTP PET Scleroderma	Supportive treatment plus plasma exchange in TTP and HUS not associated with diarrhoea. RAAS blockade for hypertensive cases and scleroderma.	
Alport's syndrome	GBM splitting and lamination	Family history. Haematuria and proteinuria with declining renal function. Boys affected in X-linked cases more severely than carrier females.	No specific treatment	ESRD in males by 3rd decade. Females affected in autosomal cases. Goodpasture's syndrome may occur following transplant due to formation of *de novo* anti-GBM antibodies.
Miscellaneous: Fibrillary GN Immunotactoid glomerulopathy Renal transplant glomerulopathy				

ANCA, anti-neutrophil cytoplasmic antibody; ESRD, end-stage renal disease; GBM, glomerular basement membrane; HUS, haemolytic uraemic syndrome; IM, immunofluorescence or immunoperoxidase microscopy; K-W, Kimmelsteil-Wilson; PET, pre-eclamptic toxaemia; RAAS, renin-angiotensin-aldosterone system; RPGN, rapidly progressive glomerulonephritis; TTP, thrombotic thrombocytopaenic purpura.

Figure 5.10 cont. Overview of secondary glomerular diseases

RPGN may be classified as either idiopathic kidney disease or as a disease secondary to other conditions such as infectious diseases, multi-system diseases, and occasionally an adverse reaction to medication. Although anti-GBM antibodies may be present along the GBM in anti-GBM disease (see below), usually there is little deposition of immune reactants such as immunoglobulin or complement within the glomerulus ('pauci-immune'). Approximately 80% of patients with active pauci-immune necrotising and crescentic glomerulonephritis have been shown to possess anti-neutrophil cytoplasmic antibodies (ANCA: Box 1), irrespective of the presence or absence of a concomitant systemic vasculitis. This strong association has allowed serological discrimination of this type of glomerulonephritis from other types of RPGN (See Figures 5.10 and 5.11).

Wegener's granulomatosis, microscopic polyangiitis and Churg-Strauss syndrome are small vessel vasculitides characterised by an association with ANCA. ANCA-associated vasculitis is the most common cause of RPGN with an incidence of 20 per million people per year and this form of kidney disease accounts for 15% of patients presenting to specialist nephrology units for RRT. The clinical picture of RPGN is often preceded by a systemic illness for several months associated with general malaise, weight loss, breathlessness, upper respiratory tract abnormalities and skin changes. Clinical examination may reveal nailfold infarcts and palpable purpura. In severe cases a renal-pulmonary syndrome supervenes, with kidney failure, alveolitis and pulmonary haemorrhage.

Since ANCA were first reported in 1982 two subtypes of ANCA have been identified, namely, cytoplasmic (c-) and perinuclear (p-) ANCA. The subtypes reflect the patterns observed by indirect immunofluorescence microscopy using alcohol-fixed neutrophils as substrate. c-ANCA is directed toward a plasma proteinase (PR3) in neutrophil primary granules and is associated with Wegener's granulomatosis, whereas the p-ANCA target antigen is usually myeloperoxidase (MPO) and is associated with microscopic polyangiitis. Autoantibodies of other specificities in rheumatoid arthritis, SLE, and inflammatory bowel disease may mimic the p-ANCA pattern, and in isolation, the finding of p-ANCA has a low specificity for vasculitis. The 'International Consensus Statement on Testing and Reporting of Antineutrophil Cytoplasmic Antibodies (ANCA)' published in 1999 was developed to optimise ANCA testing. It requires that all sera are tested by indirect immunofluorescence examination of peripheral blood neutrophils and, where there is positive fluorescence, by enzyme-linked immunosorbent assays (ELISAs) for antibodies against PR3 and MPO. Following this protocol, false positive rates of < 1% can be achieved. Testing will be further improved with standardisation and use of common ELISA units.

Box 1 Anti-neutrophil cytoplasmic antibodies (ANCA)

Laboratory investigation of vasculitic syndromes

Disease	Serological test	Antigens	Associated laboratory features
Systemic lupus erythematosus	ANA including antibodies to dsDNA and ENA (including SM, Ro [SS-A], La [SS-B] and RNP).	Nuclear antigens	Leucopenia, thrombocytopenia, Coombs' test positive. Complement activation: low serum concentrations of C3 and C4. Positive immunofluorescence using *Crithidia luciliae* as substrate. Anti-phospholipid antibodies, i.e. anti-cardiolipin, lupus anticoagulant, false positive VDRL.
Goodpasture's disease	Anti-GBM antibody	Epitope on non-collagen domain of type IV collagen.	
Small vessel vasculitis:			
Microscopic polyangiitis	p-ANCA	MPO	↑CRP
Wegener's granulomatosis	c-ANCA	PR3	↑CRP
Churge-Strauss syndrome	p-ANCA in some	MPO	↑CRP and eosinophilia
Henoch-Schonlein purpura	None		
Cryoglobulinaemia			Cryoglobulins, rheumatoid factor, complement components, hepatitis C
Medium vessel vasculitis:			
Classical PAN	None		↑CRP and eosinophilia

ANA, anti-nuclear antibodies; ANCA, anti-neutrophil cytoplasmic antibody; dsDNA, double stranded DNA; ENA, extractable nuclear antigens; GBM, glomerular basement membrane; MPO, myeloperoxidase; PAN, polyarteritis nodosa; PR3, proteinase 3; RNP, ribonucleoprotein; SM, smooth muscle; Ro (SS-A), antibodies to ENA antigen Ro (also called SS-A); La (SS-B), antibodies to ENA antigen La (also called SS-B); VDRL, venereal disease laboratory research.

Figure 5.11 Laboratory investigation of vasculitic syndromes

Highly intensive induction schedules are commenced in patients presenting with RPGN. In cases with a high index of suspicion on clinical grounds, treatment should begin empirically. The diagnosis is usually made following a kidney biopsy and the result of the ANCA or anti-GBM antibody test. High dose oral prednisolone and oral or intravenous cyclophosphamide are standard baseline treatment. Adjunctive treatments that may routinely be used in severe cases include either pulses of intravenous methylprednisolone (1 g for three days) or a series of plasma exchanges. The rationale for these approaches is to switch off production of the antibody and attenuate the proinflammatory response to tissue damage. Patients are closely followed for evidence of disease activity and signs of treatment-related toxicity for many months. Following remission of active disease drug doses are tapered and cyclophosphamide may be exchanged for azathioprine. Serial serological testing for ANCA and measurement of CRP may help decision making. Plans for long-term follow-up are made and treatment is expected to last for at least 3-5 years. Relapses may occur as immunosuppression is reduced or withdrawn. The untreated mortality of ANCA associated vasculitis is 90% at 1 year. With current management strategies the mortality rate has fallen to 20-30%. The elderly are most susceptible both to the disease and treatment-related morbidities, particularly infection. Patients that require dialysis or ventilatory support for pulmonary involvement have a higher mortality rate.

Anti-GBM disease (Goodpasture's disease) affects 0.5-1 per million people per year in the UK. Serological detection of anti-GBM antibodies is helpful to aid diagnosis in cases of RPGN. The antigens are well characterised, with the antibody directed at the α3 chain of type IV collagen. The disease is characterised by the relative lack of a prodromal illness, a very rapid deterioration in kidney function and a poor prognosis if oliguria or anuria develop. The kidney biopsy typically demonstrates crescents in all the glomeruli ('100% crescents') with each crescent at a similar stage of development. The GBM stains positively with anti-GBM antibodies using immunohistochemistry in a linear pattern. In addition to renal involvement, lung basement membrane can be affected, leading to pulmonary haemorrhage (Goodpasture's syndrome). The environment plays a critical role in determining whether anti-GBM antibodies cause lung injury since pulmonary haemorrhage only occurs in current cigarette smokers.

LUPUS NEPHRITIS

Systemic lupus erythematosus (SLE) is a chronic inflammatory disease of unknown cause that can affect the skin, joints, kidneys, lungs, nervous system, serous membranes and/or other organs of the body. The clinical course of SLE is variable and may be characterised by periods of remissions and chronic or acute relapses. Women, especially in their 20s and 30s, are affected more frequently than men. Renal involvement is termed lupus nephritis. Lupus nephritis may present variably from incidental haematuria and proteinuria, to nephrotic syndrome or a fulminating RPGN. Most patients (75%) with SLE develop abnormal urinalysis or impaired kidney function during the course of the disease. A histopathological description is required to stage the disease process in lupus nephritis. The classification of lupus nephritis has recently been revised and treatment is targeted depending on the stage of disease. In general terms, the pathological findings include a spectrum from focal mesangial proliferation to diffuse global necrotising GN. As indicated above, membranous nephropathy may also be present. Detection of lupus nephritis involves urine testing for blood and protein and tests of kidney function. In addition, serological testing for autoantibodies to nuclear antigens and measurement of complement components C3 and C4 are performed (Figure 5.11). Significant hypocomplementaemia and elevated anti-DNA titres suggest active disease. Combined use of corticosteroids and either intravenous or oral cyclophosphamide has been the conventional treatment for diffuse proliferative lupus nephritis. Treatment duration with cyclophosphamide is limited due to severe toxicity, including gonadal toxicity, haemorrhagic cystitis, bone marrow suppression and carcinogenicity. Recent data suggest that mycophenolate mofetil and corticosteroids can be an effective and well tolerated treatment alternative.

Tubulointerstitial disease

A variety of chemical, bacterial, and immunological injuries to the kidney cause either generalised or localised changes that primarily affect the tubulointerstitium rather than the glomerulus. This group of disorders is characterised by alterations in tubular function that, in advanced cases, may cause secondary vascular and glomerular damage. Interstitial nephritis, including chronic pyelonephritis, is the primary diagnosis accounting for 3.8% of incident patients onto dialysis programmes in the US. In the UK, the figure is closer to 10%. Pyelonephritis is the term associated with a bacterial infection that causes this kind of damage and is the most common of the interstitial nephritides. There are both acute and chronic types of pyelonephritis, with the acute type most commonly associated with UTI. This can develop into chronic pyelonephritis, usually as a result of a urinary tract abnormality such as abnormal urethral valves.

In addition to pyelonephritis, interstitial nephritis may present in acute or chronic forms as a result of drug toxicity or hypersensitivity (Figure 5.12). Acute interstitial nephritis (AIN) presents with ARF and may account for up to 7% of cases of ARF when an intrinsic kidney disease is diagnosed as opposed to purely toxic or ischaemic acute tubular damage. A higher incidence is observed in the elderly due to the increased incidence of drug reactions. The most common drugs are NSAIDs and β-lactam antibiotics, although over 100 different drugs have been implicated. Urinary findings may be normal or there may be low level proteinuria.

Eosinophils are often seen on light microscopy. Nephrotic syndrome may accompany an AIN associated with NSAIDs. The histopathological findings on kidney biopsy include prominent inflammation of the interstitium, with lymphocytes, polymorphonuclear cells and eosinophils being easily demonstrated. Treatment of AIN is directed at removing any causative agent. Steroids are used to promote early clinical resolution.

Sarcoidosis is a multi-system disorder associated with chronic granulomatous interstitial nephritis. Biochemical abnormalities include hypercalcaemia, hypercalciuria and elevated serum ACE, although the latter test is neither sensitive nor specific for the condition. The condition can be effectively treated with steroids.

Causes of acute interstitial nephritis	
Causes	**Examples**
Drugs (70% of cases)	NSAIDs Antibiotics: cephalosporins, penicillins, quinalones 5-aminosalicylates (e.g. mesalazine) Allopurinol Indinavir
Infections	Legionella Leptospirosis Streptococcal organisms Viruses
Autoimmune	Sjogren's syndrome (usually chronic interstitial nephritis)
Sarcoidosis (also in association with uveitis)	

Figure 5.12 Causes of acute interstitial nephritis

Renal tubular acidosis

The renal tubular acidoses (RTAs) are a diverse group of both inherited and acquired transport defects characterised by a hyperchloraemic, normal anion gap (Box 2), metabolic acidosis and urinary bicarbonate or hydrogen ion excretion inappropriate for the plasma pH. They are the result of either failure to retain bicarbonate in the proximal tubules or inability of the distal renal tubules to secrete hydrogen ions. Typically the GFR is normal, or slightly reduced and there is no retention of anions such as phosphate and sulphate, unlike in the acidosis of renal failure.

> The anion gap is a calculation describing the difference between the sums of the concentrations of the major cations (sodium and potassium) and anions (chloride and bicarbonate) in plasma. Since electrochemical neutrality is maintained, the 'gap' is of course filled by other unmeasured anions. Normal values will vary between laboratories but a range ('gap') of 14-18 mmol/L is typical. Potassium is sometimes excluded from the calculation (since it is a minor and relatively constant component) and so the normal value will be proportionally lower. In an acidosis due to loss of bicarbonate, the chloride concentration is increased, leading to a normal anion gap. In contrast, in acidosis in which other anions are increased (e.g. lactate, acetoacetate), the 'gap' is increased as anion production is generally accompanied by simultaneous decrease in bicarbonate concentration.

Box 2 The anion gap

The classification of the RTAs is based upon the biochemical expression and region of the defect rather than an understanding of the precise molecular defect. Three categories of RTA are generally recognised: distal (dRTA, type I), proximal (pRTA, type II) and that secondary to aldosterone deficiency or resistance (type IV, hyperkalaemic). A mixed proximal/distal defect can be observed in some infants and young children with primary genetic distal RTA, which was once termed 'type III RTA'. This term has been abandoned, as it is no longer considered a separate entity and indeed its frequency appears to have declined.

PROXIMAL RTA (TYPE II RTA)
pRTA is caused by impairment of proximal tubular bicarbonate reabsorption and is characterised by a decreased renal bicarbonate threshold, which is normally 26 mmol/L in adults and 22 mmol/L in children. In pRTA the threshold is lowered to ~ 15 mmol/L; once plasma bicarbonate concentration falls below this concentration, bicarbonate is reabsorbed and an acidic (pH <5.5) urine produced. pRTA may occur as a primary isolated defect or be secondary to inherited or acquired diseases, drugs or toxins that cause a Fanconi syndrome (Figure 5.13). Impaired growth is a common feature in childhood presentations of the disease but, in contrast to dRTA, nephrocalcinosis and nephrolithiasis are rarely observed. Other features of the Fanconi syndrome (e.g. glycosuria, aminoaciduria, hypokalaemia, hypophosphataemia and hypouricaemia) are commonly present.

Causes of proximal RTA (type II RTA)

Primary/secondary	Pathogenesis	Causes/notes
Primary pRTA	autosomal dominant	gene location/product unknown
	autosomal recessive	associated with mental retardation and ocular abnormalities. Caused by a defect in Na^+-HCO_3^- cotransporter NBC-1
	transient	in infancy. ?due to immaturity of the Na^+-H^+ exchanger NHE-3
Secondary pRTA	associated with the Fanconi syndrome	causes include cystinosis, galactosaemia, tyrosinaemia, hereditary fructose intolerance, Wilson's disease, Lowe's syndrome, multiple myeloma
	due to drugs/toxins	including carbonic anhydrase inhibitors (e.g. acetazolamide), aminoglycoside antibiotics, valproate, 6-mercaptopurine, lead, cadmium, mercury
	associated with other clinical entities	including amyloidosis, renal transplantation, hyperparathyroidism, nephrolithiasis, Alport's syndrome, steroid-resistant nephrotic syndrome

Figure 5.13 Causes of proximal RTA (type II RTA)

DISTAL RTA (TYPE I RTA)

Type I RTA is an inability to secrete hydrogen ions in the distal tubule and lower urinary pH maximally in the presence of a systemic acidosis. It occurs most often in infants (sometimes transiently) or young children where it is almost always observed as a primary entity (due to mutations in genes coding for specific ion transporters). However, it may also be encountered in adults, where it is more common than pRTA, and is generally secondary to a wide range of other conditions (Figure 5.14). Clinical features include a metabolic acidosis, muscle weakness, nephrocalcinosis and urolithiasis. Nephrocalcinosis and urolithiasis may be the result of decreased urinary citrate excretion secondary to cellular acidosis.

Causes of distal RTA (type I RTA)

Primary/secondary	Pathogenesis	Causes/notes
Primary dRTA	'classic' form, inherited as AD or AR or sporadic	AD form due to mutation in the gene for the Cl^--HCO_3^- exchanger AE1. AR form due to mutation in the gene for 116 kDa subunit of H^+-ATPase; this is the commonest primary form.
	AR form with deafness	due to mutations in the gene for B1 subunit of H^+-ATPase.
	with bicarbonate wasting	seen in infants and young children
	incomplete dRTA	a less severe, generally normokalaemic form with nephrocalcinosis or urolithiasis. Urinary acidification occurs at a sub-maximal rate sufficient to maintain acid-base balance (through a high rate of ammonium excretion) but ability to tolerate an acid load is compromised.
	transient	infantile form
Secondary dRTA	in the context of other inherited disorders	e.g. sickle cell disease, Ehlers-Danlos syndrome, Wilson's disease, hereditary fructose intolerance, primary hyperoxaluria type I, X-linked hypophosphataemia
	calcium disorders	e.g. primary hyperparathyroidism, magnesium-losing kidney
	dysproteinaemia	e.g. hypergammaglobulinaemia, amyloidosis, cryoglobulinaemia
	autoimmune disease	e.g. SLE, Sjogren's syndrome, chronic active hepatitis, primary biliary cirrhosis
	kidney disease	renal transplant rejection, obstructive and reflux nephropathy
	salt-retaining states	e.g. nephrotic syndrome
	drugs and toxins	e.g. amphotericin B, lithium, trimethoprim, ciclosporin

AD, autosomal dominant; AR, autosomal recessive; SLE, systemic lupus erythematosus

Figure 5.14 Causes of distal RTA (type I RTA)

The pathophysiology of the acquired secondary forms is diverse and in some cases unknown. It may occur due to changes in acid-base transporters, as in the primary forms. A so-called 'back-leak' form is described, particularly in association with certain drugs (e.g. amphotericin B), in which the kidney retains the ability to secrete hydrogen ions, but the gradient is not maintained due to back diffusion. A voltage-dependent (hyperkalaemic dRTA) form is due to failure to maintain an intraluminal negative potential and thus promote hydrogen (and potassium) ion secretion. This may be seen with urinary tract obstruction, sickle cell disease and treatment with amiloride, lithium or triamterene. This condition has many features in common with type IV RTA (see below). It is frequently associated with mild to moderate CKD. Hyperkalaemia is caused in part by the decreased GFR and partly by decreased potassium excretion relative to the filtered load.

HYPERKALAEMIC RTA (TYPE IV RTA, SELECTIVE ALDOSTERONE DEFICIENCY)
In type IV RTA there is failure of distal potassium and hydrogen ion secretion due to aldosterone deficiency or resistance. Hyperkalaemia, although mild, is a typical manifestation and causes decreased ammoniagenesis, which reduces acid excretion. Nephrocalcinosis and urolithiasis are absent in type IV RTA. Type IV RTA accompanies a large number of hyperkalaemic states and is most frequently observed in association with hypo- or pseudohypoaldosteronism (e.g. due to intrinsic renal damage or due to a range of steroid or steroid receptor synthetic defects including primary pseudohypoaldosteronism types 1 and 2). In adults, type IV RTA is normally an acquired disorder observed in the context of hyporeninaemic hypoaldosteronism as a result of chronic parenchymal renal damage (e.g. diabetic nephropathy, SLE and AIDS nephropathy) or due to drug-induced hyperkalaemia (e.g. ACE inhibitors, heparin, potassium-retaining diuretics, ciclosporin, trimethoprim, digitalis, insulin antagonists).

DIAGNOSIS OF RTA
The finding of a hyperchloraemic metabolic acidosis in a patient without evidence of gastrointestinal bicarbonate losses and with no obvious pharmacological cause (e.g. acetazolamide) should prompt suspicion of an RTA. The presence of suggestive clinical (e.g. nephrocalcinosis in dRTA) or biochemical (e.g. hypophosphataemia and hypouricaemia as a result of proximal tubular wasting in pRTA) features should also be taken into account.

In addition to plasma electrolyte measurement, preliminary investigation should include measurement of urinary pH in a fresh, early morning urine sample. The finding of a urine pH > 5.5 in the presence of a systemic acidosis supports the diagnosis of RTA. If appropriate urinary acidification cannot be demonstrated, further investigation may involve assessing the kidney's ability to excrete an acid load (furosemide or ammonium chloride load test) and reabsorb filtered bicarbonate (fractional bicarbonate excretion). These tests are described in standard clinical biochemistry textbooks.

TREATMENT OF RTA

Treatment is aimed at correcting the biochemical disturbance and, where possible, the underlying disorder, improving growth in children and avoiding the development and progression of nephrocalcinosis and CKD. In both type I and II RTAs, bicarbonate is administered to correct the metabolic acidosis. Fludrocortisone and loop diuretics may be used to treat type IV RTA.

Inherited renal disorders

Polycystic kidney disease

Autosomal dominant polycystic kidney disease (ADPKD) is the most common renal hereditary disease affecting between 1:400-1:1000 people. It accounts for 10% of the ESRD population in the UK. ADPKD can present at any age, but most commonly during adulthood. Presenting features include hypertension, haematuria, abdominal pain and UTI. A renal concentrating defect is a common feature in ADPKD. Patients without a family history may present with ESRD. It has been known for more than 100 years that this condition could be inherited as a Mendelian trait, and recently the two major genes involved in ADPKD have been identified, termed *PKD1* and *PKD2*. The *PKD1* gene is located on the short arm of chromosome 16 and codes for a 4,304 amino acid product, polycystin-1, which localises in the primary cilia of renal epithelial cells. The *PKD2* gene is located on the long arm of chromosome 4 and codes for a 968 amino acid product, polycystin-2. These proteins are involved in cell cycle regulation and intracellular calcium transport. The disease is characterised by massive enlargement of the kidneys due to cyst growth. Epithelial lined cysts arise as focal out-pouches from fewer than 5% of renal tubules. They are initially in contact with the tubular lumen and the glomerular filtrate, but the cysts detach from the parent nephron usually when greater than 2 cm in diameter.

An important observation is the highly variable clinical manifestation within families. Approximately 50% of ADPKD patients have reached ESRD by 50 years of age and 70% by 70 years. The *PKD1* and *PKD2* mutations have different prognostic implications, with *PKD2* leading to disease at a later stage than *PKD1*. ADPKD is now recognised as having extra-renal manifestations. Cysts are commonly found in the liver and pancreas. Liver involvement may be severe and require resection, although liver function is preserved. Other, non-cystic manifestations include intracranial aneurysms, mitral valve prolapse and colonic diverticulae. About 10% of ADPKD families have a strong family history of intra-cranial aneurysms. Elective surgical management is recommended for asympto-matic aneurysms > 10 mm diameter.

Individuals at risk of ADPKD may choose to undergo a diagnostic workup that includes a renal ultrasound scan. The presence of multiple bilateral cysts is required for the diagnosis. A normal USS with increasing age has a high negative predictive value with a negative scan at 20 years conferring a < 10% chance of inheritance. Mutation screening is also available. The fertility rate is similar in the ADPKD population compared to the general population and genetic counselling is recommended.

Children may present with ADPKD. Very early presentation of ADPKD can be indistinguishable from the less common autosomal recessive variant (ARPKD). The reason for the early onset is unknown. Mutation type does not correlate, however, a contiguous gene deletion of the *PKD1* and tuberous sclerosis complex 2 gene may be involved. Distinguishing ADPKD from ARPKD requires ultra-sonographic assessment of the parents. In addition, the presence of pancreatic or hepatic cysts favours diagnosis of ADPKD. A single cyst in both kidneys is adequate to make a diagnosis of ADPKD in an at-risk child. The incidence of ARPKD is 1:10,000 to 1:40,000 individuals. There is evidence that abnormalities in the primary cilia play a role in the development of ARPKD. Congenital hepatic fibrosis is a universal feature. Prenatally there may be marked kidney enlarge-ment and poor lung growth. Optimal treatment in surviving children includes supportive measures and combined liver and kidney transplantation.

Alport's syndrome (hereditary nephritis)

Hereditary glomerular diseases are being increasingly recognised. As indicated earlier, the investigation of congenital nephrotic syndromes has led to the identi-fication of mutations to key podocyte proteins such as nephrin and podocin and a greater understanding of glomerular barriers to filtration. Another condition, known as Alport's syndrome, is the result of mutations of genes coding for collagen proteins within the GBM. The primary abnormality involves the gene coding for the $\alpha 5$ chain of type IV collagen (*COL4A5*). The clinical manifestations of Alport's syndrome demonstrate that collagen proteins within other tissues are also affected, since ocular defects and sensorineural deafness are common. Alport's syndrome accounts for 1-2% of cases of ESRD and X-linked inheritance of the mutation occurs in the majority of cases (85%). Boys are therefore more severely affected, although carrier mothers may have haematuria as a result of random inactivation of one of the X chromosomes (Lyonisation). Haematuria is detected in all males and 95% of females carrying the X-linked defect. Proteinuria usually appears later and may reach the nephrotic range. Progression of disease is defined by deteriorating kidney function, proteinuria and hypertension. Diagnosis is suspected in a patient with haematuria, with or without hearing loss, and a positive family history. Confirmation requires a kidney biopsy, characterised by variable thickness of the GBM, with splitting and lamellation of the membrane in a 'basket-weave' pattern. Molecular diagnosis can be performed in patients whose family has a known genetic mutation. There is no specific treatment, although aggressive treatment of hypertension is warranted and ACE inhibitors should be used. Dialysis and transplantation are provided where appropriate. Although recurrent disease does not occur in recipients with Alport's disease who undergo kidney transplantation, an interesting and often devastating complication may occur following transplantation due to the production of antibodies to the 'new' GBM epitopes. This occurs in up to 10% of patients and can present clinically as full-blown anti-GBM disease leading to graft loss and pulmonary haemorrhage.

Inherited tubulopathies

The inherited tubulopathies comprise defects of the proximal tubule (e.g. Dent's disease, Lowe's syndrome, Wilson's disease) and transport channel defects of the loop of Henle (e.g. Bartter's syndrome) and distal tubule (e.g. Gitelman's syndrome, Liddle's syndrome, pseudohypoaldosteronism types 1a and 1b, Gordon's syndrome). They comprise a heterogeneous set of disorders often characterised by electrolyte disturbances. Many are eponymous and have been described clinically for many years; increased understanding of the molecular biology of tubular ion channel and transport pumps has now delineated the precise mechanism of disease in many of these disorders. Features of the Fanconi syndrome (glycosuria, hypophosphataemia, low molecular weight proteinuria, aminoaciduria, hypouricaemia, type II RTA) accompany disorders of the proximal tubule. In addition to electrolyte disturbances (particularly of potassium), general reasons to suspect an inherited tubulopathy include a familial disease pattern, renal impairment, nephrocalcinosis and stone formation, especially if these present at an early age. The presence of hypo- or hypertension can be an important sign in the differential diagnosis, clarification of which will often involve measurement of both plasma and urinary electrolytes in addition to measurement of renin and aldosterone. In cases where a diuretic-sensitive channel is affected, these disorders will mimic the effects of diuretic use and exclusion of covert use of diuretics is important. Some disorders may also mimic laxative abuse or surreptitious vomiting, so measurement of urinary chloride is useful in this setting. Although individually uncommon or rare, consideration of these conditions is a common reason for clinicians to seek laboratory support and advice. An awareness of these disorders is therefore critical for the clinical biochemist when considering the potential differential diagnoses in patients presenting with electrolyte imbalances. A description of Bartter's syndrome follows to illustrate the relationship between molecular defect and clinical and biochemical presentation. The main features of other tubulopathies are summarised in Figure 5.15. This section should be considered in conjunction with an understanding of tubular electrolyte handling (Chapter 1).

Inherited tubulopathies

Disorder [OMIM No]	Protein defect	Chromosome localisation	Inheritance	Clinical features/ notes	Biochemical features
Proximal tubule					
Lowe's syndrome (oculocerebral dystrophy) [309000]	OCRL1	Xq26.1	XR	hydrophthalmia, cataracts, mental retardation, hypo-reflexia, hypotonia and progressive renal failure, normotensive	Plasma: ↓K ↓CO_2 Urine: ↑LMWP ↑AA, ↑PO_4, ↑K
Wilson's disease [277900]	ATP7B	13q14.3-q21.1	AR	liver disease, neurological symptoms or both. Kayser-Fleischer rings, normotensive	Plasma:↑free copper, abnormal LFTs Urine:↑copper excretion, ↑LMWP, ↑AA ↑PO_4, ↑Glu
Dent's disease (X-linked recessive hypophosphataemic rickets) [300009]	CLCN5	Xp11.22	XR	nephrocalcinosis, nephrolithiasis, rickets or osteo-malacia, progressive renal failure, normotensive	Plasma: ↓PO_4 normal/↓K Urine: ↑LMWP, ↑AA, ↑K, ↑Ca, ↑PO_4, ↑Glu
X-linked dominant hypophosphataemic rickets [307800]	PHEX	Xp22.2-p22.1	XD	growth retardation, rickets or osteo-malacia, hypo-phosphataemia and renal defects in phosphate reabsorption and vitamin D metabolism	Plasma:↓PO_4 ↑ALP Urine:↑PO_4

Figure 5.15 Inherited tubulopathies

Disorder [OMIM No]	Protein defect	Chromosome localisation	Inheritance	Clinical features/ notes	Biochemical features
Loop of Henle					
Bartter's syndrome [601678] [241200] [607364] [602522]	NKCC2 (type I) ROMK (type II) CIC-Kb (type III, 'classic') Barttin (type IV)	15q15-q21.1 11q24 1p36 1p31	AR AR AR AR	polyuria, polydipsia muscle weakness, hypovolaemia, normo- or hypo- tensive (all types) Maternal poly- hydramnios, premature birth, perinatal salt wasting, nephrocalcinosis and kidney stones (types I and II), milder phenotype with normocalciuria (type III), sensorineural deafness, motor retardation, renal failure (type IV)	Plasma: $\uparrow$renin, $\downarrow$K, $\uparrow CO_2$, mild $\downarrow$Mg in some patients Urine: $\uparrow$Ca
Hypo- magnesaemic hypercalciuric nephrocalcinosis (magnesium- losing kidney) [248250]	PCLN1	3q27	AR	nephrocalcinosis, renal failure, ocular/ hearing defects, polyuria, polydipsia, recurrent urinary tract infections, recurrent renal colic, normotensive	Plasma: $\downarrow$Mg $\uparrow$PTH Urine: $\uparrow$Ca, $\uparrow$Mg
Distal tubule/ collecting duct					
Liddle's syndrome [177200][a]	ENaC (activating)	16p13-p12	AD	early and frequently severe hypertension, stroke	Plasma: $\downarrow$renin, $\downarrow$K, $\downarrow$Mg, $\uparrow CO_2$ Urine: $\uparrow$K
Pseudohypo- aldosteronism type Ia [264350][a]	ENaC (inactivating)	12p13, 16p13- p12	AR	presents in infancy with salt-wasting and hypotension. Cough, respiratory infections	Plasma: $\uparrow$renin, $\downarrow$Na, $\uparrow$K, $\downarrow CO_2$ Urine $\uparrow$K
Pseudohypo- aldosteronism type IIb [177735][a]	Mineralo- corticoid receptor	4q31.1	AD	presents in infancy with salt-wasting and hypotension. Milder than type Ia and remits with age	Plasma: $\uparrow$renin, $\downarrow$Na, $\uparrow$K, $\downarrow CO_2$ Urine: $\uparrow$K

Figure 5.15 cont. Inherited tubulopathies

Disorder [OMIM No]	Protein defect	Chromosome localisation	Inheritance	Clinical features/ notes	Biochemical features
Pseudohypo-aldosteronism type II (Gordon's syndrome) [145260]	Unknown (?WNK)	1q31-q42 12p13 17q21-q22	AD	hypertension, muscle weakness, short stature, intellectual impairment. Correction of the biochemical abnormalities by thiazide diuretics.	Plasma: ↓ renin, ↑K, ↓CO_2, ↑Cl Urine: ↓ K
Gitelman's syndrome [263800]	NCCT	16q13	AR	hypotension, weakness parasthesia, tetany, fatigue and salt craving Presentation generally much later in life than Bartter's and hypo-calciuria is typical. Biochemically can mimic thiazide use.	Plasma: ↑renin, ↓K, ↓Mg, ↑CO_2 Urine: ↓calcium: creatinine ratio (useful in distinguishing Gitelman's and Bartter's).
X-linked nephrogenic diabetes insipidus type I [304800]	V2 receptor	Xq28	XR	hyperthermia, polyuria, polydipsia, dehydration, inability to form concentrated urine, mental retardation if diagnosis delayed. Symptoms in infancy.	Hyperosmolar plasma, dilute urine
Autosomal dominant nephrogenic diabetes insipidus type II [192340]	AQP2	12q13	AD and AR	polyuria, polydipsia, dehydration, inability to form concentrated urine. Symptoms after first year of life.	Hyperosmolar plasma, dilute urine

AA, aminoaciduria; AD, autosomal dominant; AR, autosomal recessive; Glu, glucose; LMWP, low-molecular weight protein-uria; OMIM, Online Mendelian Inheritance in Man; XD, X-linked dominant; XR, X-linked recessive.

[a]see Figure 1.6

Figure 5.15 cont. Inherited tubulopathies
A useful resource for further information is the Online Mendelian Inheritance in Man™ (OMIM) web-site (www.ncbi.nlm.nih.gov/entrez/query.fcgi?db=OMIM).

Bartter's syndrome
This is a group of autosomal recessive disorders typically presenting antenatally or neonatally and characterised by renal salt wasting, polyuria, polydipsia, impaired urinary concentrating ability and a hyperreninaemic, hypokalaemic metabolic alkalosis. Mild hypomagnesaemia is seen in some patients.

Biochemically the effects resemble those of loop diuretic use, but clinically the phenotype is highly variable. This arises because the syndrome encompasses inactivating mutations affecting at least four different transporters/channels in the loop of Henle. The biochemical effects are predictable from knowledge of the function of these transporters and channels (Figure 1.5).

Mutations in the genes encoding NKCC2 (type I) or ROMK1 (type II) are associated with a severe phenotype, including maternal polyhydramnios (probably due to excessive urine production *in utero*), premature birth, life-threatening salt-wasting in the perinatal period and hypercalciuria. Patients with ROMK1 defects tend to have less severe hypokalaemia. Nephrocalcinosis is almost universal.

The milder ('classic', type III) Bartter's syndrome is due to defects in the basolateral pump, CLC-Kb. Although the phenotype is extremely variable (neonatal, life-threatening presentations do occur), these patients typically present in the first year of life with weakness and hypovolaemia and normal urinary calcium excretion. Nephrocalcinosis and kidney stone formation are not usually present.

A fourth type (Barttin, type IV) has been described due to a mutation in barttin, a protein that acts as an essential activator subunit for the renal chloride channel CLC-Ka in addition to CLC-Kb. This is a severe phenotype with intrauterine onset, profound renal salt and water wasting, renal failure, sensorineural deafness and motor retardation.

Treatment of Bartter's syndrome includes the use of potassium supplements, spironolactone and NSAIDs.

Inherited metabolic diseases

Many inherited metabolic diseases affect the function of the kidney or are characterised by excessive urinary excretion of an intermediary metabolite(s). Most are generalised disorders affecting other organs in the body and having renal sequelae as a systemic secondary consequence of the underlying disorder (e.g. due to vomiting). Figure 5.16 lists disorders that have a major effect on kidney function. In some cases, kidney disease occurs as a result of accumulation of an intermediary metabolite (e.g. galactose 1-phosphate in galactosaemia) whereas in others the disorder occurs due to failure of a transport mechanism (e.g. cystinuria). Some of these disorders appear relatively benign (e.g. iminoglycinuria). The renal effect often manifests as Fanconi syndrome as described above. An overview of all of these disorders is beyond the scope of this book. Cystinosis and Fabry's disease are described below as examples. Cystinuria is described in more detail later in this chapter.

Inherited metabolic diseases with major renal manifestations	

Disorder	OMIM number
Adenine phosphoribosyltransferase deficiency	102600
Alport's syndrome	104200
Cystinosis	219800
Cystinuria	220100
Galactosaemia	230400
α-galactosidase A deficiency (Fabry's disease)	301500
Glycogenosis type I (von Gierke's disease)	232200
Hartnup's disease	234500
Hereditary fructose intolerance	229600
Hereditary xanthinuria	278300
Hyperuricaemic nephropathy (familial juvenile gout)	162000
Hypoxanthine-guanine phosphoribosyltransferase deficiency	308000
Iminoglycinuria	242600
Lecithin cholesterol acyltransferase deficiency	245900
Lysinuric protein intolerance	222700
Phosphoribosyl pyrophosphate synthetase superactivity	311850
Primary hyperoxaluria type I	259900
Primary hyperoxaluria type II	260000
Tyrosinaemia type I	276700
Wilson's disease	277900

Figure 5.16 Inherited metabolic diseases with major renal manifestations.
Note, this list is not exhaustive. A useful resource for further information is the Online Mendelian Inheritance in Man™ (OMIM) web-site which may be searched using the OMIM numbers given in the figure
(www.ncbi.nlm.nih.gov/entrez/query.fcgi?db=OMIM).

CYSTINOSIS

This is a rare, autosomal recessive disease caused by defective export of cystine across the lysosomal membrane as a result of inactivating mutations in cystinosin, an integral lysosomal membrane protein. There is cellular accumulation of cystine with crystallisation that destroys tissues. Classic cystinosis presents in the first year of life with failure to thrive, polyuria, polydipsia, hypophosphataemic rickets and other features of Fanconi syndrome. Progressive renal damage generally results in renal failure by 10 years of age. Diagnosis relies upon measurement of the cystine concentration of peripheral leucocytes or cultured fibroblasts. While treatment with dialysis and transplantation (the disease does not recur in the donor kidney) has improved outcome, there are several extrarenal complications, including blindness, pancreatic failure, primary hypogonadism and neurologic deterioration. Treatment with cysteamine, which depletes lysosomal cystine, slows the rate of progression of renal disease and also improves the ocular complications.

FABRY'S DISEASE

This is an X-linked inborn error of glycosphingolipid metabolism due to deficiency of the lysosomal enzyme α-galactosidase A. The disease presents with haematuria and proteinuria and in males usually progresses to renal failure by the fifth decade. Female carriers may be affected. Glycosphingolipid accumulates particularly in vacuoles in the podocyte, giving the cytoplasm a foamy appearance. Other renal and extrarenal cells are also affected. The diagnosis is established by measuring α-galactosidase A activity in plasma or peripheral leucocytes. Treatment involves the use of recombinant human α-galactosidase A replacement therapy in addition to dialysis and transplantation. Glycosphingolipid accumulation does occur in allografts, but does not appear to cause graft failure.

Toxic nephropathy

Anatomical, physiological and biochemical features make the kidney susceptible to insult from a variety of medicinal and environmental agents. Factors contributing to the sensitivity of the kidney include its large blood flow, concentration of filtered solutes during urine production and the presence of a variety of xenobiotic transporters and metabolising enzymes. Toxic nephropathy commonly occurs either as a result of decreased renal perfusion, due to precipitation within the tubule or due to direct toxic effects on the proximal tubule. In some cases, the conjugation of environmental chemicals (e.g. mercury and cadmium) to glutathione and/or cysteine targets these chemicals to the kidney where inhibition of renal function occurs through a variety of mechanisms that are not completely understood. Renal injury induced by chloroform is dependent on renal cytochrome P450 metabolism to toxic metabolites. Other compounds, such as paraquat and diquat, damage the kidney via the production of reactive oxygen species. While some drugs can cause kidney damage in the presence of normal renal function, a far greater variety of drugs can cause problems in patients with kidney disease, predominantly due to accumulation as a result of decreased renal elimination. The British National Formulary (www.bnf.org) has an appendix devoted to prescribing issues in the presence of renal impairment. A list of drugs and environmental toxins known to cause kidney damage is given in Figure 5.17. Both glomerular and tubulointerstitial damage result from exposure to these toxins; detection of both requires biochemical monitoring of GFR/serum creatinine concentration and tubular and glomerular proteinuria.

Toxic nephropathy: causes, pattern and markers

Compound category	Drug/toxin	Type of renal injury/ pathology	Biomarkers/notes
Antibacterial agents	aminoglycosides (e.g. neomycin, gentamicin, tobramycin, amikacin)	nonoliguric ARF	plasma: ↓K, ↓Mg, ↓Ca urine: ↑LMWP, ↑Glu nephrotoxicity major and common side effect
	amphotericin	initially distal tubular injury followed by medullary injury	plasma: ↓K, ↑creatinine dRTA
Antiviral/antiprotozoal agents	acyclovir	nonoliguric ARF due to tubular obstruction and interstitial inflammation	crystalluria and haematuria
	pentamidine	tubular toxicity	plasma: ↓Mg, ↓Ca urine: ↑Mg, ↑Ca
	indinivar	nephrolithiasis, irreversible RF in some patients	crystalluria and haematuria
Radiocontrast agents	e.g. iothalamate, iodixanol	oliguric or nonoliguric RF, generally reversible. Proximal tubular damage	by definition, ↑plasma creatinine > 44 μmol/L from baseline after contrast administration
Drugs used in transplantation	ciclosporin	acute reversible and chronic irreversible nephrotoxicity. ↓RBF, glomerular vasculopathy and interstitial fibrosis	dRTA, impaired urinary concentrating ability
	tacrolimus	↓RBF and interstitial fibrosis	nephrotoxicity less common than with ciclosporin
Antitumour drugs	cisplatin	irreversible dose-related and cumulative RF. TIN with heavy proteinuria. Often ARF.	urine: ↑Mg, ↑PO$_4$, tubular casts with ↑LMWP in early stages
	methotrexate	nonoliguric ARF. Tubular atrophy and interstitial inflammation	only seen in association with high dose therapy
	interleukin-2	reversible ARF due to ↓RBF	observed in 90% of cases of high dose therapy

Figure 5.17 Toxic nephropathy: causes, pattern and markers

Compound category	Drug/toxin	Type of renal injury/ pathology	Biomarkers/notes
Other drugs	ACE inhibitors	dramatic ↓GFR due to ↓efferent arteriolar tone	especially in the setting of bilateral renal artery stenosis. ↑plasma creatinine and K
	5-aminosalicylic acid (e.g. mesalazine olsalazine)	occasional ATN and irreversible kidney damage	tubular proteinuria
	cyclooxygenase-2 inhibitors	probably a similar pattern of renal injury to NSAIDs (see below)	
	lithium	distal tubular damage with nephrogenic diabetes inspidus ± dRTA	
	penicillamine	membranous glomerulopathy with NS, occasionally ARF	proteinuria
	NSAIDs	several forms of nephropathy identified including: haemo-dynamically-mediated ARF, TIN ± NS, salt and/or water retention, hyperkalaemia, CKD/ESRD ('analgesic nephropathy')	depends on type of effect
Heavy metals	cadmium	subtle but irreversible TIN	Fanconi syndrome with RTA. ↑urinary metallothionein
	gold	membranous glomerulopathy but normal GFR maintained	proteinuria < 3.5 g/24h
	lead	proximal tubular atrophy with interstitial fibrosis	reversible Fanconi syndrome in children with poisoning. In lead workers, urinary proteinuria < 2 g/24h in association with ↑plasma urate, hypertension ± gouty arthritis

Figure 5.17 cont. Toxic nephropathy: causes, pattern and markers

Compound category	Drug/toxin	Type of renal injury/ pathology	Biomarkers/notes
Heavy metals (cont.)	mercury	proximal tubular damage with ATN	urine: ↑LMWP
Other environmental agents	hydrocarbons (e.g. paints, dry cleaning solvents)	ATN, chronic TIN, glomerulonephritis	tubular proteinuria ± ↑plasma creatinine
	paraquat	ATN secondary to ↓RBF due to shock and direct toxic effects of paraquat	↑plasma creatinine

ACE, angiotensin converting enzyme; ARF, acute renal failure; ATN, acute tubular necrosis; dRTA, distal renal tubular acidosis; ESRD, end stage renal disease; GI, glycosuria; LMWP, low-molecular weight proteinuria; NS, nephrotic syndrome; NSAIDs, non-steroidal anti-inflammatory drugs; RBF, renal blood flow; RF, renal failure; TIN, tubulointerstitial nephropathy

Figure 5.17 cont. Toxic nephropathy: causes, pattern and markers

Monoclonal light chains and kidney disease

Immunoglobulin (Ig) molecules are formed in secretory B cells (plasma cells) from polypeptide heavy (H) and light (L) chains. The chains are linked covalently by disulphide bonds. Each chain has a constant and a variable region. The heavy chains α, β γ, δ, and ε, denote the antibody isotype, whereas light chains are peptide molecules that are called kappa (κ) and lambda (λ). A complete Ig molecule will contain either κ or λ. The proportion of Ig containing κ versus λ is 3:2 in humans. The molecular weight of light chains is around 22.5 kDa. There is an excess of light over heavy chains resulting in the release of free light chains into the circulation. In normal individuals, the small quantity of circulating polyclonal free light chains is filtered by the glomerulus and around 90% is reabsorbed in the proximal tubule. Light chains are then degraded by proteases and the amino acids returned to the circulation. When the concentration of filtered light chains increases, proximal tubule cell damage may occur. Light chains can deposit in the kidney as casts, fibrils and precipitates or crystals, giving rise to a spectrum of disease including myeloma cast nephropathy, AL-amyloidosis and light chain deposition disease (LCDD). Light chains may cause tubular dysfunction, especially of the proximal tubular cells (Fanconi syndrome). Characteristically, the light chain variable domain is resistant to degradation by proteases in lysosomes within the tubular cells and therefore they accumulate. Clinical features include RTA and phosphate wasting.

Myeloma

Myeloma or 'multiple myeloma' is a neoplastic proliferation of plasma cells that produce excessive amounts of monoclonal Ig (paraprotein), so-called M protein, which gives rise to the characteristic peaks in serum protein electrophoresis on agarose gel. The clone of plasma cells proliferates in the bone marrow and often results in extensive skeletal destruction with osteolytic lesions, osteopenia, and/or pathological fractures. Other common clinical findings include anaemia, hypercalcaemia, and renal insufficiency. The clonal proliferation is associated with either an excess of whole immunoglobulin, or pure light chain production. In multiple myeloma, complete monoclonal Igs (usually IgG or IgA) are accompanied in the plasma by variable concentrations of free light chains that appear in the urine as BJP.

Light chains are not detected by urinary dipsticks, which primarily measure albumin. Urine should be examined for the presence of BJP by sensitive laboratory immunophoretic and immunofixation techniques in any patient with acute or chronic kidney disease of uncertain cause. These methods can identify M proteins and light chains in the serum and/or the urine in 98% of patients with myeloma. Recently developed assays that can measure serum free κ and λ light chains are likely to have an increasing role in the diagnosis and monitoring of myeloma, but at present the clinical utility of these assays has not been unequivocally established. Immune paresis, with reduction in non-paraprotein Ig, is characteristic of myeloma. In some cases (non-secretory myeloma) it is not possible to detect a serum paraprotein or urine BJP.

The incidence of myeloma is 40 new cases per million population per year. An apparent reported increase in incidence recently is probably related to enhanced availability and use of medical facilities, especially by older people. Myeloma is more common in men than women and the median age at presentation is 65 years. Impairment of kidney function at presentation occurs in almost 50% of patients. Typical precipitants of kidney failure include dehydration, hypercalcaemia, infection, and nephrotoxic drugs such as NSAIDs and radiocontrast media. Approximately 10% of patients have severe renal involvement caused by the direct effects of light chains on the kidney as a result of deposition of intact light chains within tubules in association with THG. This is termed myeloma cast nephropathy (or myeloma kidney). The condition is characterised by ARF and the kidney biopsy typically demonstrates tubular obstruction by numerous fractured casts and tubule cell inflammation (Plate 12).

Treatment of kidney failure in myeloma has two main objectives. Firstly, supportive therapy is targeted at the known predisposing factors for cast nephropathy and secondly, the production of light chains from the malignant B cell clone is reduced following chemotherapy. Supportive therapy includes increased fluid intake where permissible to 3 L/day, treatment of hypercalcaemia, treatment of infection and withdrawal of NSAIDs. Chemotherapy protocols vary between centres but usually include combination chemotherapy with cytotoxic agents such as cyclophosphamide and adriamycin, along with the potent steroid, dexamethasone. Recently, the anti-angiogenic drug, thalidomide, has been used to induce remission in some patients. In addition to chemotherapy, several sessions of plasma exchange within the first week of diagnosis of kidney failure in myeloma reduces the free light chain load. However, the evidence of the clinical benefit of plasma exchange is conflicting. A multi-centre trial (MERIT) is underway in the UK to identify whether plasma exchange is a useful adjunct to chemotherapy. However, data from a large Canadian trial suggest that in patients with ARF at the onset of myeloma, plasma exchange does not significantly reduce the composite outcome of death or dialysis dependence at 6 months.

General supportive measures in myeloma include treatment of anaemia with blood products and the use of erythropoiesis stimulating agents (ESAs) such as erythropoietin. Autologous bone marrow transplantation is considered in some cases of myeloma and if successful, improves life expectancy significantly. Poor prognostic features include dialysis-dependent kidney failure, increased β_2-microglobulin, C-reactive protein, and lactate dehydrogenase concentrations, along with abnormal cytogenetics (especially deletion of 13q). Bone lesions are treated with bisphosphonates and palliative radiotherapy may be required for painful lesions.

As discussed above, myeloma cast nephropathy is characterised by glomerular filtration of *intact* light chains and subsequent tubular damage. Excess production of monoclonal light chains (or, rarely, heavy chains) can cause disorders in which *fragments* are deposited in the kidney and other tissues: AL-amyloid, LC- and HC-deposition diseases (LCDD and HCDD).

AL-amyloid
Primary or systemic (AL) amyloidosis is a clonal plasma cell proliferative disorder in which fibrils of monoclonal light chains are deposited in the kidney and other tissues (such as the liver, heart, and peripheral nervous system). Approximately 10 percent of patients have multiple myeloma. In AL-amyloid, the circulating light chains are taken up by macrophages and partially metabolised. Light chain fragments are then secreted from the macrophages, and these fragments can precipitate to form the characteristic Congo red positive, β-pleated fibrils. In 75% of cases the fibrils are derived from λ light chains. Amyloid was first described 150 years ago and the term was coined because the tissue deposits resembled plant starch. Congo red staining (leading to green birefringence with

polarised microscopy) was introduced in the 1920s. AL-amyloid can occur alone or in association with multiple myeloma or, much less often, Waldenstrom's macroglobulinaemia or other lymphoproliferative disorders such as lymphoplasmacytic lymphoma.

AL-amyloid is a common cause of nephrotic syndrome in patients aged 60 years and over. The diagnosis of AL-amyloid can be suspected from the clinical findings of nephrotic syndrome and the presence of a serum or urinary paraprotein. However, 10-15% of patients with primary amyloid do not have a detectable serum or urinary paraprotein and a bone marrow sample may be necessary to identify a clonal expansion of plasma cells. Although the presence of amyloidosis may be suggested by the history and clinical manifestations (e.g. nephrotic syndrome in a patient with multiple myeloma), the diagnosis must be confirmed by tissue biopsy. Biopsy of a clinically involved site is suggested for patients with a limited number of affected organs. Therefore, a kidney biopsy should be performed if nephrotic syndrome is an isolated finding (Plate 13). Fat pad aspiration biopsy is sensitive at demonstrating amyloid in patients with multiorgan involvement and may be a safer option for patients with more than one organ involved. The involvement of multiple organs can be demonstrated non-invasively using a radiolabelled serum amyloid protein (SAP) scan. Treatment options include chemotherapy to reduce production of monoclonal proteins and bone marrow transplantation. In the setting of decreased production of light chains following chemotherapy there may be repair of organ damage or slowing of progression of organ damage.

Light-chain deposition disease (LCDD)
LCDD typically presents as nephrotic syndrome and/or renal insufficiency. Most patients with renal involvement progress to ESRD requiring dialysis. Less frequently, liver involvement can occur with hepatomegaly and liver dysfunction, either alone or in combination with renal involvement. Rarely, LCDD may involve the heart and lead to cardiomyopathy and heart failure. Patients may progress to overt multiple myeloma; some patients may have multiple myeloma at initial diagnosis. LCDD is pathogenetically similar to AL-amyloid except that the light chain fragments do not form fibrils and the deposits are Congo red negative. The deposits in LCDD are usually granular and composed of κ-light chains. The constant region of the light chain is typically deposited in this disorder and immunostaining is strongly positive. Both AL-amyloid and LCDD have a poor prognosis and the mean survival is 18 months, with 50% of patients dying from cardiac failure.

Renal stone disease

Nephrolithiasis, the formation of kidney stones or calculi, can occur in the renal pelvis, the ureter or the bladder. In developed countries bladder stones are now uncommon, as the causative factors of malnutrition and infection have been eliminated. Calcification can also occur throughout the parenchyma (nephrocalcinosis). Kidney stone formation is often considered to be a nutritional or environmental disease, linked to affluence, but genetic or anatomical abnormalities are also significant. Approximately 10% of the population of the Western world are thought to have formed at least one kidney stone by the age of 70 years. For most stone types there is a male preponderance. The passage of a stone is associated with severe pain called renal colic; this may last for 15 minutes to several hours and is commonly associated with nausea and vomiting. There is some evidence that stone formation contributes to the development of CKD.

Urine contains many mineral salts that are present in concentrations that approach, and may exceed, their solubility products. Crystals can form spontaneously if the salt concentrations are high enough, or, alternatively, preformed nuclei can provoke their formation. Human urine contains a number of promoters (e.g. sodium, oxalate and urate) and inhibitors (e.g. citrate, magnesium) of stone formation, the concentrations of which can be influenced by dietary and metabolic factors. The predominant risk factor is poor hydration, concentrated urine increasing the concentrations of the mineral salts and predisposing to crystallisation. In addition to identifiable specific inherited diseases (e.g. cystinuria), stone formation occurs on a background of genetic risk, the details of which are poorly understood. The majority of kidney stones found in the Western world are composed of one or more of the following substances: calcium oxalate with or without phosphate (frequency 67%), magnesium ammonium phosphate (12%), calcium phosphate (8%), urate (8%), cystine (1-2%), and complex mixtures of the above (2-3%). These poorly soluble substances crystallise within an organic matrix, the nature of which is not well understood.

Initial diagnosis and investigation of stones requires radiological investigations to explore the degree of intrarenal calcification and papillary damage. Plain X-rays are undertaken at initial presentation, although it should be noted that urate and other purine stones and some cystine stones are radiolucent. An intravenous urogram or spiral CT scan may be performed to establish the presence and extent of urinary tract obstruction, intrarenal reflux and ureteric dilation. Further investigation of the patient with kidney stones or suspected of being a stone former involves analysis of blood, urine and of the stone itself, should one be obtained.

Small stones (≤ 5 mm in diameter) often pass spontaneously in the urine as 'gravel'. Although surgical treatment to remove large staghorn calculi may still be necessary, the commonest form of treatment is ultrasonic extracorporeal shock wave lithotripsy (ESWL), which can be applied to stones between 5 mm and 2 cm in diameter. Following treatment and successful removal of a stone, follow-up monitoring is required, as many patients will have recurrent disease. In the absence of medical treatment the recurrence rate may be as high as 50% at 10 years.

The cornerstone of disease management remains adequate fluid intake. However, specific management of disease depending on the metabolic abnormality present is also important. Further investigation of stone formers may be guided by knowledge of the type of stone formed. However, the increasing use of lithotripsy means that there is often no stone material available for analysis and management is based upon knowledge of the blood and urinary composition (Figure 5.18).

Typical 'metabolic screen' undertaken in stone formers

Serum
sodium, potassium, chloride, bicarbonate, creatinine, calcium, phosphate and urate

24 h urine
volume and 24 h urinary excretion of calcium, magnesium, phosphate, oxalate, urate, creatinine, sodium and citrate

Fresh early morning urine sample
microbiology (to exclude infection) and measurement of urinary pH and cystine

---

Figure 5.18 Typical 'metabolic screen' undertaken in stone formers. Metabolic evaluation should be undertaken at least six weeks after the episode of renal colic and should ideally be done on several occasions. It is most informative when undertaken on an outpatient basis with patients pursuing their normal diet and lifestyle.

When available, analysis of the chemical constituents of stones may be useful. It complements and guides metabolic investigation of the patients and may be particularly useful in identifying rare stone types (e.g. xanthine, dihydroxyadenine), artefacts (e.g. Munchausen syndrome) or the identification of drugs precipitating in the urinary tract (e.g. triamterine, indinavir). Conversely, it has been argued that stone analysis is not useful clinically since the stone material passed often does not represent the initial metabolic derangement. This is due to the phenomenon known as epitaxy, whereby non-specific stone material, typically arising as a result of urinary tract infection (e.g. struvite) may accumulate on a pre-existing 'metabolic' nidus, the latter of which may not be detected during stone analysis. A variety of stone analysis techniques have been used over the years with infrared spectroscopy generally being preferred. It must be emphasised that the qualitative methods of analysis that have been used in many laboratories over the years have poor specificity and sensitivity.

Calcium stones

The majority of stones formed in the Western world are composed of calcium, most commonly in association with oxalate, although calcium phosphate and urate may also be present, either alone or in combination with calcium oxalate. As a consequence, urinary calcium measurement has been the central investigation. However, the significance of the role of oxalate is increasingly being appreciated and this has resulted in changes to the optimal management of hypercalciuria. As a rough guide, calcium oxalate stones tend to suggest hyperoxaluria as the main cause while calcium phosphate stones suggest hypercalciuria and/or failure to adequately acidify urine. Hypercalciuria, daily excretion in excess of 0.1 mmol/kg body weight, is the most common metabolic abnormality seen in calcium stone formers, being observed in up to 50% of patients.

Traditionally, investigation focused on whether patients demonstrated hypercalciuria while fasting ('renal hypercalciuria') or in response to a calcium load ('absorptive hypercalciuria'). Patients with absorptive hypercalciuria have abnormally high intestinal calcium absorption compared with non-stone formers (possibly due to a relative increase in $1,25(OH)_2D_3$ concentrations and/or changes in intestinal vitamin D receptor activity). Formerly, treatment in these patients focused on dietary restriction of calcium intake, but this is now generally regarded as ineffective and actually counterproductive, since it results in an increase in intestinal oxalate absorption and increased risk of stone formation. At least a subset of patients with renal hypercalciuria are now thought not to have a renal transport defect, but to have increased turnover of skeletal calcium. Patients with hypercalciuria are known to have reduced bone mineral density and dietary calcium restriction may exacerbate a tendency to osteopenia/osteoporosis.

A more useful approach is to classify hypercalciuria as being either hypercalcaemic or normocalcaemic. The former is most commonly due to primary hyperparathyroidism, which is seen in approximately 5% of stone formers. Normocalcaemic causes of hypercalciuria constitute the majority and are generally classified as idiopathic (although specific causes such as renal tubular acidosis, high sodium intake and prolonged immobilisation should be excluded). Idiopathic hypercalciuria is probably a combined syndrome of a range of intestinal and skeletal abnormalities in calcium metabolism. In addition to increasing fluid intake, idiopathic hypercalciuric patients appear to benefit from a diet that is low in animal protein and sodium. High sodium excretion as a result of high consumption inhibits tubular reabsorption of calcium, with a consequent increase in the risk of calcium stone formation. Sodium is easily and cheaply measured in urine and represents a modifiable risk factor. Other therapeutic manoeuvres that may be useful include pharmacological modification of renal calcium handling using thiazide diuretics, alkaline citrate and reducing oxalate and increasing fibre intake.

OXALATE

Oxalate is an end product of metabolism, predominantly derived from breakdown of glyoxylate and glycine. Its plasma concentration is 11-27 μmol/L and it is excreted in the urine at a rate of 200-400 μmol/24 h. Less than half of urinary oxalate is derived directly from dietary sources. Intestinal oxalate absorption is increased when the availability of calcium in the intestine is reduced. Hyperoxaluria is a powerful promoter of calcium oxalate stone formation. It may occur as a result of excessive dietary intake, malabsorption and/or steatorrhoea (enteric hyperoxaluria) or an inborn error of metabolism (primary hyperoxaluria).

Enteric hyperoxaluria commonly occurs in association with inflammatory bowel diseases and may contribute to an increased incidence of stone formation in such patients. Fat malabsorption contributes to the formation of calcium soaps, increasing the enteric concentration of unbound oxalate that is absorbed through the damaged bowel wall. Primary hyperoxaluria may be type 1 (glycollic aciduria) or type 2 (L-glyceric aciduria). Patients with type 1 disease present in the first decade of life with recurrent calcium oxalate nephrolithiasis. Inheritance is autosomal recessive and survival is poor. Type 2 disease is rarer and has been claimed to run a milder course, despite the passage of similarly high concentrations of urinary oxalate. The urinary excretion of oxalate may increase to 700 μmol/24 h when a diet containing an excess of oxalate-rich foods is taken and to as much as 3 mmol/24 h in patients with primary hyperoxaluria.

Ideally, urine for oxalate analysis should be collected into acid to prevent the formation of calcium oxalate crystals. This also prevents *ex vivo* formation of oxalate from ascorbate, a cause of factitious hyperoxaluria in individuals ingesting excessive amounts of vitamin C. A dietary history is important in the evaluation of calcium oxalate stone formers. Patients who are excreting large amounts of oxalate may be offered dietary advice to modify their risk of future stone formation. Foods rich in oxalate include beetroot, spinach, sorrel, almonds, wheat bran, strawberries, rhubarb, blackcurrants, peanuts and chocolate. Patients may also be treated with calcium carbonate, which binds oxalate in the gut rendering it unavailable for absorption. Alternatively, pyridoxine (vitamin B_6) can be used; this increases the catabolism of oxalate to more soluble products. It should be remembered that the use of calcium-lowering diets, once favoured in the treatment of calcium stone formers, increases intestinal absorption of oxalate.

MAGNESIUM

Magnesium forms complexes with oxalate that are more soluble than calcium oxalate, therefore inhibiting stone formation. Administration of magnesium has been shown to reduce enteral calcium absorption and has been proposed as a treatment for idiopathic hypercalciuric stone formers. However, oral magnesium supplementation may have unpleasant side effects, including diarrhoea, and a positive benefit in terms of reducing stone recurrence has not been demonstrated.

URATE

Urate may potentiate calcium stone formation, although this is not universally accepted. At high urinary pH, colloidal sodium urate may promote calcium oxalate crystallisation. Hyperuricosuria is common in calcium stone forming patients and treatment with allopurinol, which decreases urate synthesis, reduces the stone recurrence rate. Allopurinol treatment is therefore recommended for hyperuricosuric patients with calcium stone disease. The formation and management of pure urate stones is discussed below.

CITRATE

Urinary citrate inhibits stone formation by forming soluble complexes with calcium. It is present in the diet in many fruits. Excretion (typically 1-5 mmol/24h) is reduced in the calcium stone forming population. Urinary citrate measurement may be of value in the assessment of stone forming risk, particularly in the setting of dRTA where the reduction in filtered bicarbonate appears to increase tubular reabsorption of citrate with consequent hypocitraturia. Inadequate urinary acidification compounds the increased risk of calcium stone formation. Treatment with carbonic anhydrase inhibitors (e.g. acetazolamide) mimics dRTA with consequent increase in stone risk. Hypocitraturia may also be seen in malabsorption and UTI. Administration of oral alkaline citrate increases urinary citrate concentration by increasing the pH of tubular cells. It has been shown to be effective in the treatment of nephrolithiasis, although there are side effects, it is unpalatable and compliance is poor.

Urate stones

Pure uric acid stones account for approximately 8% of all urinary tract stones and, unlike many of the calcium-containing stones, are radiolucent. Although serum and urinary uric acid should be measured in stone formers, many uric acid stone formers do not demonstrate either hyperuricosuria or hyperuricaemia. However, this may reflect the use of reference intervals derived in a purine-rich, Westernised society. The aetiology of uric acid stone formation also involves the passage of a persistently acid urine with loss of the postprandial alkaline tide. Undissociated uric acid (pK_a 5.57) is relatively insoluble, whereas urate at pH 7.0 is > 10 times more soluble. Thus, in patients with urinary pH persistently < 6.0, normal urinary concentrations of uric acid will produce supersaturation. This goes some way towards explaining why patients with ileostomies, who produce a concentrated, acidic urine, are particularly prone to uric acid stone formation. Allopurinol and alkalinisation with potassium alkali salts, to maintain a urinary pH of approximately 6.5, are the mainstays of treatment of uric acid stones. However, hyperuricosuria is also a risk factor for calcium stone formation (see above) and it is therefore important to avoid increasing the urinary pH above 7.5.

Cystine stones

Cystinuria is an autosomal recessive condition in which there is excessive urinary excretion of cystine due to a defect in proximal renal tubular reabsorption. This arises due to inactivating mutations in one of the two possible subunits (rBAT or $b^{0+}AT1$) of the renal multisubstrate basic amino acid transporter. In the commonest form of the disease there is therefore also excess excretion of the dibasic amino acids (lysine, ornithine and arginine) although their presence in excess in urine appears benign. (N.B. Cystinuria should not be confused with cystinosis, in which there is excess urinary excretion of cysteine due to a systemic abnormality – see above).

The normal urinary excretion of cystine is 40 to 400 μmol/24 h. Its relatively low limit of solubility (1250 μmol/L) is exceeded in many patients with cystinuria, resulting in the formation of hexagonal crystals and, ultimately, cystine stones. Cystinuria may present at any age from infancy to old age, although presentation is commonest in the second and third decades.

The finding of a cystine stone should prompt confirmation of cystinuria by urinary analysis. It could be argued, however, that all stone formers should be screened for cystinuria; at least 10% of cystinurics form stones in which cystine cannot be detected, presumably due to epitaxy. The index of suspicion should be increased in patients who are relatively young stone formers and in those with a positive family history. Once a cystinuric patient is diagnosed, it is important to screen all members of the family, particularly to detect affected siblings.

In the first instance, treatment is aimed at maintaining cystine below its saturation point (i.e. by maintaining high fluid intake, particularly at night). Other treatments include urinary alkalinisation (cystine is more soluble in alkaline urine) and chelation with D-penicillamine, alpha-mercaptopropionylglycine, or captopril.

Struvite ('infection') stones

Struvite (also called triple phosphate or infection) stones are composed of magnesium ammonium phosphate hexahydrate. The formation of such stones requires chronic, recurrent UTI with urea splitting organisms (e.g. *Proteus* sp.) and such stones are therefore commoner in females and in certain patient populations, e.g. those with paraplegia. An underlying anatomical predisposition is also often present. The risk of progression to CKD appears higher in patients who develop infection related stones than in other forms of stone disease.

Further reading

DIABETIC NEPHROPATHY
American Diabetes Association. Nephropathy in diabetes. Diabetes Care 2004; **27(suppl.1):** S79-83.

Gross JL, de Azevedo MJ, Silveiro SP, Canani LH, Caramori ML, Zelmanovitz T. Diabetic nephropathy: diagnosis, prevention, and treatment. Diabetes Care 2005; **28:** 176-88.

Schena FP, Gesualdo L. Pathogenetic mechanisms of diabetic nephropathy. J Am Soc Nephrol 2005; **16(suppl.1):** S30-33.

HYPERTENSION AND THE KIDNEY
Moser M, Setaro JE. Clinical practice: resistant or difficult-to-control hypertension. N Engl J Med 2006; **355:** 385-92.

GLOMERULAR DISEASES
Barratt J, Feehally J. IgA Nephropathy. J Am Soc Nephrol 2005; **16:** 2088-97.

Eddy, AA. Nephrotic syndrome in childhood. Lancet 2003; **363:** 629-39.

Pozzi C, Andrulli S, Del Vecchio L, Melis P, Fagazzi GB, Altieri P *et al.* Corticosteroid effectiveness in IgA nephropathy: long-term results of a randomised control trial. J Am Soc Nephrol 2004; **15:** 157-63.

Savige J, Davies D, Falk RJ, Jennette JC, Wiik A. Antineutrophil cytoplasmic antibodies and associated diseases: a review of the clinical and laboratory features. Kidney Int 2000; **57:** 846-62.

TUBULOINTERSTITIAL DISEASE / PYELONEPHRITIS
Baker RJ, Pusey CD. The changing profile of acute tubulointerstitial nephritis. Nephrol Dial Transplant 2004; **19:** 8-11.

RENAL TUBULAR ACIDOSIS
Soriano JR. Renal tubular acidosis: the clinical entity. J Am Soc Nephrol 2002; **13:** 2160-70.

INHERITED RENAL DISORDERS
Sayer JA, Pearce SHS. Diagnosis and clinical biochemistry of inherited tubulopathies. Ann Clin Biochem 2001; **38:** 459-70.

Toxic nephropathy
Palmer BF, Henrich WL. Toxic Nephropathy. In Brenner and Rector's The Kidney, 7th edition, Chapter 34, Saunders, Philadelphia, 2004.

Monoclonal light chains and kidney disease
Kyle RA, Rajkumar SV. Multiple myeloma. N Engl J Med 2004; **351:** 1860-73.

Merlini G, Bellotti V. Molecular mechanisms of amyloidosis. N Engl J Med 2003; **349:** 583-96.

Renal stone disease
Moe OW. Kidney stones: pathophysiology and medical management. Lancet 2006; **367:** 333-44.

Chapter 6

Complications of kidney disease

Cardiovascular disease

Cardiovascular disease is the commonest cause of death among patients with kidney disease and such deaths occur at a younger age than among the background population. The incidence of cardiovascular disease is 7 to 10-fold greater in patients with CKD than in non-CKD age and gender matched controls. Indeed, the majority of CKD patients die from cardiovascular disease before they progress to kidney failure. Even after stratification by age, gender, race, and the presence or absence of diabetes, cardiovascular mortality in dialysis patients is 10 to 20 times higher than in the general population (Figure 6.1). The spectrum of cardiovascular disease in CKD includes heart failure, ischaemic heart disease, arrhythmia, valvular disease and peripheral vascular disease. Structural heart diseases, such as left ventricular hypertrophy (LVH) and valvular heart disease, are very common in CKD.

Cardiovascular disease mortality

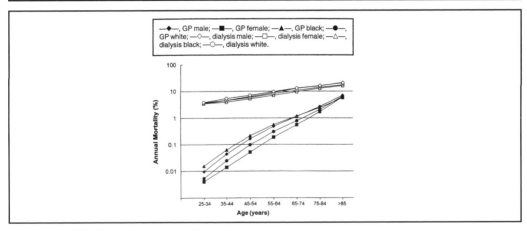

Figure 6.1 Cardiovascular disease mortality defined by death due to arrhythmias, cardiomyopathy, cardiac arrest, myocardial infarction, atherosclerotic heart disease, and pulmonary oedema in the general population (GP) (Data from National Centre for Health Statistics, US, multiple cause of mortality data files) compared to ESRD treated by dialysis. Data are stratified by age, race and gender. Note the logarithmic scale. From Foley RN, Parfrey PS, Sarnak MJ. Clinical epidemiology of cardiovascular disease in chronic renal disease. Am J Kidney Dis 1998; **32 (suppl 3):** S112-S119 with permission.

Observational studies have indicated that cardiovascular disease occurs at an early stage in CKD. Microalbuminuria and proteinuria are also independently associated with increased risk of cardiovascular disease and cardiovascular mortality. These associations may arise because CKD causes an elevated level of cardiovascular disease, or because cardiovascular disease causes CKD, or because some other factors, such as diabetes or hypertension, cause both CKD and cardiovascular disease.

Most clinical consequences of cardiac disease result from cardiomyopathy or ischaemic heart disease. In addition to atherosclerosis, vessels may be damaged by arteriosclerosis due to sustained haemodynamic overload and by vascular calcification. The relative contribution of each of these processes to cardiac dysfunction in CKD varies from patient to patient.

Left ventricular hypertrophy

LVH is an adaptive process that occurs in response to a long-term increase in myocardial work caused by LV pressure or volume overload. The haemodynamic risk factors comprising pressure overload include arterial hypertension, arteriosclerosis (increased arterial wall stiffness) and aortic stenosis. Those comprising volume overload include increased extracellular volume, anaemia and arteriovenous fistulae. Pressure overload contributes to concentric hypertrophy whereas volume overload causes eccentric hypertrophy. However, volume and pressure factors are rarely discrete and one often contributes to the effects of the other. Pressure and volume overload also result in adaptive arterial hypertrophy and remodelling. Initially, these can be viewed as normal physiological responses to increased cardiac demand (e.g. as seen in trained athletes), but under uraemic conditions the process becomes maladaptive with a sustained imbalance between energy expenditure and production, resulting in chronic energy deficit, myocyte death and arteriosclerosis. At autopsy, hearts from dialysis patients are often enlarged with grossly thickened walls and a dilated LV cavity. There is myocyte hypertrophy and hyperplasia of the non-myocytic components.

LVH is present in over 70% of patients commencing dialysis and a significant proportion of patients with earlier stages of CKD; the proportion of patients with LVH increases as kidney function declines. In the dialysis population it is an independent predictor for cardiac death. Increasing age, increased systolic blood pressure, presence of diabetes and decreased haemoglobin concentration are independent predictors of LVH in the CKD population. The significance of anaemia as a secondary complication of CKD is considered elsewhere in this chapter, but its importance in the setting of LVH appears paramount. Anaemia has both direct and indirect effects on left ventricular function and growth, which overall cause a chronic increase in cardiac output and work. A fall in blood haemoglobin concentration of 1 g/dL increases risk of LVH by 6%; returning haemoglobin concentration to normal is possible and may have cardiovascular benefits.

Heart failure

Heart failure occurs when the ventricular muscle is incapable of maintaining sufficient output to meet the metabolic demands of the body. The clinical presentation classically includes dyspnoea and pulmonary venous congestion due to increased pulmonary capillary pressure. Among the dialysis population this presentation can also occur due to pure volume overload in the absence of cardiac failure. Both LVH and coronary artery disease are risk factors for the development of heart failure, the prevalence of which among dialysis patients exceeds 30%. Most dialysis patients with LVH will have some impairment of LV diastolic function, characterised by clinical heart failure with preserved systolic function. Filling of the left ventricle during diastole may be affected by heart rate, ventricle muscle compliance (stiffness) and atrial contraction. Systolic dysfunction (diminished myocardial contractility) is also common, either due to the presence of ischaemic heart disease or sustained biomechanical stress (due to prolonged and marked haemodynamic overload) or both. In practice, discrimination between diastolic and systolic dysfunction is difficult because of the coexistence of multiple pathologies. Echocardiographic assessment of ventricular function and filling is helpful to characterise the type of cardiac failure. If the left ventricle end-diastolic volume is large, this is suggestive of systolic failure; if it is small diastolic dysfunction predominates. In the presence of heart failure, a variety of mechanisms are brought into play in an attempt to maintain ventricular output. These include increased secretion of hormones such as angiotensin II, arginine vasopressin and natriuretic peptides.

Ischaemic heart disease

Among patients treated by dialysis, the prevalence of coronary artery disease, characterised by critical stenoses of the major coronary arteries, is approximately 40%. In the setting of LVH, a significant percentage of dialysis patients also have non-atheromatous ischaemic heart disease, in which the increased myocardial oxygen demand cannot be met.

Risk factors for cardiovascular disease in CKD

The risk factors for cardiovascular disease in CKD are a mixture of the traditional and CKD-specific. Traditional risk factors such as diabetes, hypertension and dyslipidaemia are more prevalent in CKD patients. In addition there are a number of putative risk factors that are CKD-related (Figure 6.2). The role of some of these risk factors is considered below.

Risk factors for cardiovascular disease in CKD

Traditional risk factors*	Non-traditional risk factors
Older age	Extracellular fluid overload
Male gender	Proteinuria
Hypertension	Anaemia
Left ventricular hypertrophy	Abnormal calcium and phosphate metabolism
Increased LDL cholesterol	Dyslipidaemia (abnormal lipoprotein profile)
Decreased HDL cholesterol	Electrolyte imbalance
Diabetes mellitus	Infection
Smoking	Thrombogenic factors
Sedentary lifestyle	Oxidative stress
Menopause	Increased homocysteine
Family history	Uraemic toxins
	Inflammation
	Malnutrition

LDL, low density lipoprotein; HDL, high density lipoprotein; CKD, chronic kidney disease

*Some of the traditional risk factors are more prevalent, or more severe, among the CKD population.

Figure 6.2 Traditional and non-traditional risk factors for cardiovascular disease in CKD

DYSLIPIDAEMIAS

Various dyslipidaemias are associated with CKD and the prevalence of dyslipidaemia is high. The pattern of dyslipidaemia in CKD differs from that seen in non-CKD. It is characterised by an accumulation of partly metabolised triglyceride-rich particles (predominantly very low density lipoprotein (VLDL) and intermediate density lipoprotein (IDL) remnants), mainly due to abnormal lipase function. This causes hypertriglyceridaemia and low concentrations of HDL-cholesterol. Although total cholesterol concentration may be normal, there is often a highly abnormal lipid subfraction profile with a predominance of atherogenic, small, dense LDL particles. Lipoprotein (a) concentrations are also increased in CKD.

There are no large, prospective studies examining the relationship between cardiovascular disease and dyslipidaemia in ESRD patients. Randomised controlled trials of the effects of lipid-lowering therapy on cardiovascular mortality and kidney function have, to date, excluded patients with CKD. Several such studies are currently underway, e.g. the SHARP trial but, pending the results of these studies, the NICE CKD guidelines (see Chapter 8) have recommended that lipid management in patients with CKD should follow the Joint British Societies' recommendations, despite the fact that it is explicitly stated in these that the cardiovascular risk prediction charts should not be used for patients with renal dysfunction.

HYPERTENSION
Hypertension is prevalent at all stages of CKD and is an independent risk factor for LVH, heart failure and ischaemic heart disease. Hypertension may either cause or be the result of CKD, or both. Hypertensive nephropathy is discussed in Chapter 5.

DIABETES
The presence of diabetes in CKD patients predicts both coexistence, extent and progression of cardiovascular disease. In particular, diabetic CKD patients have an increased burden of LVH. Excessive cardiovascular mortality in diabetic dialysis patients appears to be mediated via ischaemic heart disease rather than progression of LVH.

INFLAMMATION
Many studies have now shown a relationship between CRP and cardiovascular mortality in CKD. The cause of increased CRP concentrations in CKD patients is unclear but may include back-filtration of endotoxin during dialysis, vascular access, unrecognised infection and bio-incompatibility of peritoneal dialysate.

HOMOCYSTEINE
Patients with CKD have an excess prevalence of mild-to-moderate hyperhomocysteinaemia, which has been independently linked to the development of cardiovascular disease in observational studies. There is as yet little evidence that intervention to reduce homocysteine concentrations affects the risk of disease in the general population or in CKD patients. However, correction of folate deficiency is considered good clinical practice in CKD patients.

VASCULAR CALCIFICATION AND PHOSPHATE MANAGEMENT

Calcification of vascular structures is associated with a number of conditions, including cardiovascular disease and ESRD. Calcium phosphate deposition, in the form of bioapatite, can occur in blood vessels, myocardium and heart valves. Calcified deposits are found in distinct layers of the blood vessels, related to the underlying pathology. Calcification of the major arteries occurs along the intimal lining of blood vessels in association with atheroma. However, in CKD (and also in diabetes and with increased age) medial and adventitial calcification may also occur, reducing the compliance of the vessel (vascular stiffening and arteriosclerosis). Intimal and medial calcification may occur independently or in association with each other.

It has been known for over 100 years that patients with kidney failure have vascular calcification; this is a mixture of intimal and medial (atheromatous and arteriosclerotic) calcification. Vascular calcification has been studied in both CKD and non-CKD populations using modern sophisticated imaging. Electron-beam computed tomography acquires serial sections of the aortic arch, the coronary vessels and the aorta. Areas of calcification can be identified and allocated a calcium score (Agatston Score). This approach cannot distinguish between intimal or medial calcification but, in non-CKD patients, the score correlates with atherosclerotic plaque burden, plaque instability and risk of myocardial infarction. Once considered a relatively benign observation in association with ageing and atheroma, it is now thought that calcification may itself initiate and promote cardiovascular disease, particularly in the setting of CKD. Decreased vascular compliance removes the cushioning effect of the major arteries during cardiac contraction, leading to so-called increased pulse wave velocity and pulse pressure. This causes rebound pulse waves to return more quickly to the heart (increased afterload) during the cardiac cycle, contributing to LVH and compromised coronary perfusion.

Dialysis patients as young as 20 years exhibit vascular calcification, decades before it would be anticipated in the non-CKD population. In the ESRD population, increasing evidence supports a link between vascular calcification and cardiovascular risk and, in turn, between hyperphosphataemia/increased serum calcium-phosphate product (calculated by multiplying the concentrations of calcium and phosphate) and both calcification score and cardiovascular risk. Thus, deranged calcium and phosphate metabolism is now considered a major non-traditional risk factor for cardiovascular disease in CKD.

Recent studies have explored the molecular pathophysiology of vascular calcification. A number of proteins that are inhibitors of calcification, including matrix gamma-carboxyglutamic acid (Gla) protein, are constitutively expressed by vascular smooth muscle cells in normal media but are down-regulated in calcified arteries. In calcified plaques, vascular smooth muscle cells express osteoblast-like gene expression profiles, as demonstrated by *in situ* hybridisation. The presence of bone proteins such as osteocalcin, suggests that osteogenesis also plays a role in vascular calcification. The identification of natural inhibitors of calcification in plasma, such as human fetuin-A (AHSG or α_2-Heremans Schmid glycoprotein), suggests that the vascular endothelium may be continually subjected to calcification stresses and that regulatory systems break down in uraemia. AHSG concentrations are significantly lower in plasma of haemodialysis (HD) patients than in healthy controls. Increased calcium-phosphate product promotes apatite nucleation and crystal growth and would be expected to exacerbate vascular calcification by any of the above mechanisms, in addition to having other direct effects on vascular cells that promote mineralisation.

Hyperphosphataemia and increased calcium-phosphate product (the major component of which is the phosphate concentration) are associated with increased mortality in ESRD patients. The relative risk of death in the US for those HD patients with serum phosphate concentration > 2.10 mmol/L is 1.27 relative to those with serum phosphate concentrations of 0.77 to 2.10 mmol/L. In at least 50% of HD patients, the serum phosphate concentration is > 1.94 mmol/L and in 25% of patients it is > 2.32 mmol/L. The mainstays of ESRD management include reduction of hyperphosphataemia and normalisation of low serum calcium concentration, which results from decreased 1-α hydroxylase activity. For example, the UK Renal Association standard for pre-dialysis serum phosphate concentration is 1.1 to 1.8 mmol/L. Strategies include dietary restriction of phosphate intake, the use of phosphate binders to restrict intestinal absorption and the use of vitamin D and vitamin D analogue supplements. Phosphorus is consumed in many foods and is linearly associated with protein ingestion. The recommended daily allowance is reduced for patients on dialysis to around 800 mg. Treatment with vitamin D analogues increases gut absorption not only of calcium, but also of phosphorus, from 60-70 % to almost 85%. The use of phosphate binders, which are consumed with meals, is almost universal in dialysis patients and reduces phosphorus absorption to 30-40%.

The emerging risks associated with vascular calcification are driving a rethink of management in this area. Phosphate binders have largely been calcium (or aluminium) containing and calcium based binders are associated with increased risk of calcification. However, studies using the non-calcium, non-aluminium-containing phosphorus binder, sevelamer hydrochloride, in HD patients have shown significant attenuation in the rate of calcification of vessels. Patients were also less likely to develop hypercalcaemia although there was a tendency to worsening acidosis. The hope for future studies is that attenuation (and possibly reversal) of vascular calcification will improve patient survival.

Cardiac biomarkers and kidney disease

The biochemical diagnosis of myocardial infarction in patients with ESRD has always been problematic. Commonly, increases in the cardio-specific form of creatine kinase, CK-MB, are observed in the absence of myocardial infarction. This is attributed to production and release of CK-MB from regenerating skeletal muscle, consequent upon the myopathy associated with ESRD. Early in the evaluation of cardiac troponins (cTn) as markers of cardiac disease, it became apparent that serum troponin concentrations (particularly cardiac troponin T, cTnT) are also commonly increased in patients with ESRD, even in the absence of an acute coronary event. The significance of this observation has been the subject of considerable debate and remains a barrier to universal acceptance of cardiac troponins as specific markers of cardiac damage. This is an important limitation given the preponderance of cardiovascular disease in patients with kidney disease. Initially this observation was attributed to non-specific binding and re-expression of cTnT in the skeletal muscle of uraemic patients. This view was reinforced by the fact that increased serum cardiac troponin I (cTnI) concentrations were less commonly observed in ESRD and that detection of cTnI in uraemic patients appeared to demonstrate better specificity for myocardial infarction, as defined clinically.

Later modifications of the cTnT assay show decreased cross-reactivity with the skeletal isoform, but the observation of increased concentrations of cTnT in the serum of patients with ESRD persists. Depending on the cut-off chosen, between 20% and 90% of patients with ESRD have increased serum cTnT concentrations. Subsequently, elevation of both cTnT and cTnI concentrations has been demonstrated in patients with kidney disease and the variable reports of cTnT compared to cTnI have been attributed to problems with the sensitivity, diagnostic threshold and standardisation of the latter assay. This view is supported by recent studies using cTnI assays with improved sensitivity.

The possibility that increased cTn concentrations reflect decreased clearance or analytical interference from uraemic serum has not been definitively excluded but is unlikely on the basis of pre- and post-dialysis study results and that the observation is not universal amongst uraemic patients. It is increasingly accepted that the cTn detected in serum from patients with ESRD is derived from myocytes and is present in the same form as that seen in patients who have suffered an acute coronary syndrome (ACS). This could result from sub-clinical myocardial ischaemic release of troponin, myocardial remodelling in the development of LVH or as a result of uraemic pericarditis or myocarditis. Perhaps the strongest arguments supporting the reality of increased cTn concentrations in this setting are the associations that have now been demonstrated with poor outcome (mortality), in both the ESRD and non-dialysis CKD populations.

The use of cardiac troponins to diagnose ACS in the general population has revolutionised management. Unfortunately, it has failed to simplify the diagnosis of ACS in patients with ESRD. In non-uraemic patients, an increased serum cTn concentration in the presence of ischaemic symptoms and/or characteristic electrocardiogram (ECG) changes is generally considered sufficient evidence to satisfy the diagnosis. In the setting of ESRD, this is clearly not the case and there is considerable clinical confusion as to how the diagnosis can be established in such patients. Diagnosis of ACS in ESRD is complicated by the fact that such patients are at higher risk of silent myocardial ischaemia and atypical clinical presentations. In addition, a previous history of angina is often absent. ECG investigations are also difficult to interpret; abnormalities such as left bundle branch block and left ventricular strain patterns are extremely common, making evaluation difficult. Consequently ACS may be missed or there may be a significant delay in diagnosis. This, coupled with an apparent reluctance to use aspirin, β-blockers, thrombolytic therapy or to refer patients with moderate renal insufficiency for angiography or angioplasty, may partly explain the significantly higher mortality seen in this group. In a recent study, one year mortality following myocardial infarction was 24% in patients with normal renal function compared to 66% in patients with kidney disease (serum creatinine 220-345 μmol/L).

A great deal more work is needed to determine the usefulness of cardiac troponins as clinical tools in patients with suspected ACS and kidney disease. While a negative cTn concentration is clearly useful in this setting, management problems arise in ESRD patients with a suspected ACS who have an increased cTn concentration. In the absence of a simple gold standard diagnostic test for ACS, clinical and cardiovascular specific outcomes studies in this population will hopefully provide the evidence base for the development of useful management guidelines.

Given the high prevalence of LVH and heart failure in patients with CKD, there is considerable interest in the use of B-type natriuretic peptide (BNP) and its N-terminal fragment (N-terminal pro-B-type natriuretic peptide, NT-proBNP). These peptides are co-secreted from myocytes as a result of ventricular stretch arising in part from fluid overload. In the non-CKD population they have been found to be useful biomarkers of heart failure. In the setting of CKD, increased serum concentrations of BNP and NT-proBNP have been observed, as would be expected given the preponderance of heart disease, and relationships have been observed between their concentrations and left ventricular mass. However, concentrations of both BNP and, particularly, NT-proBNP (which relies upon glomerular filtration for its clearance) appear to be increased as a consequence of declining GFR, irrespective of cardiac hormone output. This markedly reduces their specificity for heart failure. Notwithstanding this, both natriuretic peptides appear to have high predictive value for mortality among patients with kidney disease.

Cardiac disease develops early in the course of CKD. Although tests to assess cardiac function and diagnose heart disease in asymptomatic patients are available (in the form of cardiac echocardiography, myoview scans and exercise ECGs), for health economic reasons they are not offered to all CKD patients. The ability to detect cardiac disease at an early stage could facilitate aggressive and focussed treatment of those at increased risk. Many of the traditional cardiac risk factors, as well as those specifically or more commonly associated with renal disease (i.e. LVH, anaemia and hyperparathyroidism [see below]) can be modified by aggressive therapy. This does, however, require early identification of patients at increased risk of cardiac disease. It is the hope that cardiac biomarkers could be used to screen for cardiovascular risk in CKD patients and facilitate targeted early intervention.

Renal osteodystrophy and secondary hyperparathyroidism

Pathogenesis of renal bone disease

Evidence of hyperparathyroidism and abnormalities of bone mineral homeostasis are seen early in CKD and inevitably progress as CKD worsens. Apart from the musculoskeletal abnormalities, so-called 'renal osteodystrophy', there are effects on soft tissue calcification that may account for much of the morbidity and mortality of these patients; these have been discussed above. In advanced CKD, morphological changes may occur in the bone and cause clinical symptoms and increase the risk of bone fractures, particularly non-vertebral bone fractures. The term 'renal osteodystrophy' refers to the alteration of bone morphology in patients with CKD and is quantifiable on bone biopsy. The components used to classify renal osteodystrophy include turnover and mineralisation. Turnover reflects the rate of skeletal remodelling, which is normally the coupled process of bone resorption and bone formation. This is usually an active and continuous process. Mineralisation reflects how well bone collagen becomes calcified during the formation phase of skeletal remodelling. The cells that are responsible for new bone formation are osteoblasts recruited from bone marrow mesenchymal cells. These cells release alkaline phosphatase (ALP). In contrast, large multinucleated osteoclasts are cells that 'eat away' at bone, causing resorption of mineral from the bone matrix. PTH is the major regulator of bone turnover and skeletal cellular activity.

Normal mineral metabolism is characterised by a complex homeostatic system that exists to maintain plasma calcium concentrations within 2% of normal. The system comprises sensing tissues such as the parathyroid glands, calciotropic hormones (PTH and activated vitamin D [calcitriol]) and effector tissues upon which the hormones act (kidney, bone and intestine). The parathyroid gland cells have a calcium-sensing receptor (CaSR) on the surface of the cell membrane. The calcium-sensing receptor belongs to the family of G-protein-coupled receptors. The ligand is inorganic Ca^{2+} and, once stimulated by calcium within the receptor, downstream signals inhibit production of PTH within the parathyroid cell. If the plasma calcium concentration falls, the CaSR is not stimulated permitting PTH gene transcription and translation to occur with subsequent secretion into the blood. PTH is released from the parathyroid glands predominantly as an 84 amino acid peptide (PTH(1-84)). Classic biological activity, mediated via interaction with the PTH receptor PTH1R, resides in the N-terminus of the molecule. C-terminal (C-PTH) fragments are also directly secreted by the parathyroid gland. Following release, PTH(1-84) undergoes proteolytic degradation in Kupffer cells in the liver; the resulting C-PTH, but not N-terminal fragments, may re-enter the circulation. The variously derived PTH fragments and PTH(1-84) are then excreted renally.

Secreted PTH acts on the kidneys via PTH1R in several ways. Firstly, calcium is actively reabsorbed by the renal tubules. Secondly, phosphate is excreted by the renal tubules (phosphaturic effect). Thirdly, PTH upregulates the enzyme 1-α hydroxylase and increases renal conversion of vitamin D to the active form (calcitriol: 1,25-dihydroxy vitamin D_3). Activated vitamin D increases calcium absorption from the intestine and bone thus attempting to return plasma calcium concentration to normal. PTH also acts on the skeleton causing calcium and phosphate to be released into the blood.

As kidney function declines, elevated concentrations of PTH are observed. PTH begins to rise as the GFR falls below 70 mL/min/1.73 m^2. Significant secondary hyperparathyroidism develops at a GFR $<$ 45 mL/min/1.73 m^2. There is a complex interplay of factors leading to secondary hyperparathyroidism but it is the tendency to develop hypocalcaemia that stimulates increased PTH secretion. Hypocalcaemia develops because as the GFR falls, phosphate is retained, causing a reduction in ionised calcium. High phosphate concentrations can also directly stimulate the parathyroid glands to increase PTH production in CKD (Figure 6.3).

A further mechanism involved in the development of secondary hyperparathyroidism in CKD is calcitriol deficiency. Calcitriol is produced by renal proximal tubular cells and as CKD progresses there is reduced production, beginning as GFR falls below approximately 45 mL/min/1.73 m^2. Calcitriol acts as an inhibitor of PTH secretion via the vitamin D receptor (VDR) in the parathyroid cell. There is good evidence that the expression of the VDR and CaSR is reduced with progression of secondary hyperparathyroidism and parathyroid hyperplasia. The VDR is a 427 amino acid peptide and is widely found in tissues including parathyroid glands, intestine and osteoblast-like cells.

Phosphate in the pathogenesis of secondary hyperparathyroidism
• Phosphate induced hypocalcaemia • Phosphate induced decrease in calcitriol concentrations • Direct stimulatory effect of phosphate on PTH secretion • Decreased skeletal response to PTH due to hyperphosphataemia

Figure 6.3 Phosphate retention in the pathogenesis of secondary hyperparathyroidism

The normal ionised calcium concentration is approximately 1.2 mmol/L. At this concentration, secretion of PTH from the parathyroid glands is 25% of its maximal value. The relationship between PTH and calcium is characterised by an inverse sigmoidal curve and hypocalcaemia causes a very rapid increase in PTH. Reduced CaSR expression, as in CKD, affects the sensitivity of parathyroid cells to extracellular calcium. As secondary hyperparathyroidism develops, the sensitivity of the parathyroid cells to calcium diminishes. Severe secondary hyperparathyroidism is associated with hyperplasia of the glands and ultimately nodular hyperplasia. These grossly enlarged glands tend to be resistant to medical therapies for secondary hyperparathyroidism as they have significantly reduced expression of both the CaSR and VDR.

Increased resistance to N-terminal PTH has been proposed as a mechanism in the pathogenesis of adynamic bone disease (Figure 6.4). It has been suggested that this may be due to accumulation of C-PTH fragments [mainly PTH(7-84)] as kidney disease progresses. A range of *in vitro* and *in vivo* studies have demonstrated biological activities of C-PTHs including PTH(7-84) that would tend to oppose those of the intact hormone. These actions are presumably mediated via PTH receptors other than PTH1R. The importance of these actions in the evolution of adynamic bone disease is still unclear, but it has been suggested that ratios of PTH(1-84) to PTH(7-84) could be used to assess and stage low bone turnover as an alternative to bone biopsy. Recent studies have failed to support the initial enthusiasm for this approach. Although PTH(7-84) may possess biological activity as an antagonist to PTH(1-84), any clinical role in the assessment of renal osteodystrophy remains to be confirmed.

Clinical investigation of renal osteodystrophy

Plain X-ray films provide minimal information in the evaluation of renal osteody-strophy in the majority of CKD patients. Exceptions are advanced forms of bone disease such as severe osteitis fibrosa cystica (sub-periosteal erosions) and osteo-malacia (Looser zones). However, radiographs remain an important part of the evaluation of renal osteodystrophy in children with CKD.

Traditionally, the characteristic lesions seen in renal osteodystrophy have been defined by the histological appearance of bone following biopsy. A bone biopsy taken from the iliac crest of the pelvis may be subjected to tetracycline labeling techniques to assess bone turnover. The individual is requested to ingest tetracy-cline for 2-3 days and, following an interval of 10-14 days, a further, different tetracycline is administered. Tetracycline drugs are taken up into bone and dynamic measurements of osteoblast function can be made following labeling of the biopsy material with appropriate fluorochromes.

Bone biopsies are rarely undertaken in UK nephrological practice and the emphasis for understanding and recognition of renal bone disorders has been placed almost entirely on measurement of biochemical markers of bone turnover, in particular plasma calcium, phosphate, ALP and PTH. The most common forms of renal osteodystrophy are attributable largely to variations in the plasma concentrations of PTH and are summarised in Figure 6.4. As such, circulating PTH concentration has been used as a surrogate marker of bone turnover and is used to diagnose and guide treatment of renal osteodystrophy.

Historically, dialysis water contained high concentrations of aluminium. In addi-tion, the commonly used oral phosphate binder, aluminium hydroxide, led to concerns regarding aluminium toxicity in dialysis patients. Evidence of toxicity was demonstrated by bone biopsy with features of osteomalacia or adynamic bone disease and direct staining for aluminium. Quantities of aluminium in dial-ysis water are now much lower due to changes made to the general water supply as well as the treatment that dialysis water receives in the renal unit plant. Nevertheless, in patients treated with aluminium hydroxide, monitoring for aluminium toxicity remains mandatory.

Classification of renal bone disease

Type of bone disease	Description	Pathogenesis
High-turnover		

Osteitis fibrosa	Increased bone resorption
	Disorganised woven
	  (non-lamellar) collagen
	  deposition
	Increased osteoid
	Increased rate of bone formation
		Secondary hyperparathyroidism

Low-turnover		
Osteomalacia	Decreased osteoid formation Aluminium accumulation often present Decreased bone formation rate	Excess aluminium Vitamin D deficiency Acidosis Lack of trace elements
Adynamic or aplastic bone	Few remodelling sites Low bone formation rate Decreased osteoid deposition	Low PTH concentration Resistance to N-terminal PTH Excess aluminium Older patients Diabetes Peritoneal dialysis
High and low-turnover		
Mixed disease		Secondary hyperparathyroidism Aluminium Unknown factors

Figure 6.4 Classification of renal bone disease

Measurement of PTH in CKD

Measurement of PTH in the presence of renal impairment has always been problematic. In the 1970s it became apparent that PTH radioimmunoassays cross-reacted with C-PTH fragments that accumulated in the presence of renal failure. The development of a two-site immunoassay (Nichols Allegro immunoradiometric assay [IRMA]) in the 1980s, described as an 'intact' PTH assay, seemed to resolve this issue. However, in the mid-1990s it was realised that intact PTH assays cross-reacted to a large degree with a C-PTH fragment thought to be PTH(7-84) and other less prevalent fragments of PTH that accumulated in renal failure. Cross-reactivity with this fragment probably accounts for approximately 50% of immunoreactive PTH in patients with ESRD, although the exact degree of cross-reactivity varies between methods. Many manufacturers continue to market their assays as 'intact' PTH assays, although it is clear that they lack specificity.

Results using second generation PTH assays do not agree among kidney disease patients, either with each other or with the original Nichols Allegro IRMA; among dialysis patients, commonly used commercial assays may over- or under-estimate PTH by up to 50% compared with the Nichols Allegro IRMA. Between-method variability is due to a variety of factors, including lack of common standardisation, variation in recovery of PTH(1-84) and differences in the extent of cross-reactivity with PTH(7-84)(Figure 6.5).

Variability of PTH results using commercial PTH assays

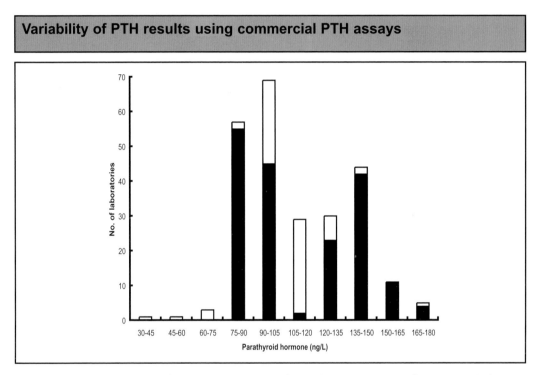

Figure 6.5. Variability of plasma PTH results using a variety of commercial PTH assays. The sample was pooled ethylenediaminetetracetic acid plasma (Seracare, California, USA) supplemented (240 parts in 700 parts) with a pooled plasma obtained from patients with renal failure. The histogram shows results for all methods. The solid boxes indicate results obtained from laboratories using Roche ElecSys methods, whereas hatched boxes indicate DPC Immulite methods. Data supplied by and reproduced with permission from UK NEQAS (Edinburgh, distribution 95, September 2006).

In the last few years, PTH assays have become available that claim to measure only PTH(1-84). These third generation assays utilise polyclonal antibodies targeted to epitopes on the first few N-terminal amino acids. Unfortunately, these third generation assays are not yet widely available on automated platforms suitable for the majority of laboratories. There is a tight correlation between second and third generation assays across a range of PTH concentrations and the clinical advantages of using third generation assays have yet to be clearly demonstrated. However, it is likely that these assays will be used more widely in the future.

Management of renal osteodystrophy

A variety of strategies are employed to manage renal osteodystrophy (Figure 6.6). Medical management particularly focuses on amelioration of the hyperphosphataemia that drives secondary hyperparathyroidism. Active vitamin D replacement in a variety of forms is widely used to treat both hypocalcaemia and secondary hyperparathyroidism. However, treatment is complicated by the development of hypercalcaemia and hyperphosphataemia due to increased VDR expression in the intestine with increased absorption of calcium and phosphate from the gastrointestinal tract. Surgical parathyroidectomy is reserved for refractory cases.

A range of guidelines relating to the management of renal osteodystrophy are now available. In addition to plasma calcium and phosphate concentrations, guidelines often use plasma PTH concentration as a therapeutic target and decision threshold. It should be borne in mind that the somewhat limited evidence correlating renal bone disease and plasma PTH concentrations upon which guidelines have been based relates largely to experience with second generation 'intact' assays, in particular the prototype Nichols Allegro IRMA. The validity of these targets and decision limits when transferred to other PTH assays is therefore questionable.

For dialysis and renal transplantation patients, the UK Renal Association standard states that the PTH concentration should be more than twice and less than four times the upper limit of normal of the assay. Using this cut-off requires that the upper limit of normal is accurate and appropriate for the assay used which is often not the case; a UK NEQAS survey in July 2005 indicated that the majority of participants were using an upper limit of normal close to 65 ng/L (6.9 pmol/L), irrespective of the known variations in recovery of the assays used. If a concentration is to be used as a target value, then it would seem desirable to recognise the effect of assay bias and to set assay-specific cut-offs. However, in the US, the NKF-K/DOQI has proposed a single upper target for dialysis patients of <300 ng/L (31.8 pmol/L), irrespective of the PTH assay used.

Treatment of secondary hyperparathyroidism in CKD

Therapy	Drugs	Side effects	Comments
Dietary control of phosphate		May be restrictive and unpalatable	Difficult to attain since phosphate in many foods
Ensure adequate dialysis			Three times a week haemodialysis is inadequate to normalise phosphate in the majority of cases. Daily short-hours dialysis is associated with normal or low phosphate. Daily short-hours or nocturnal haemo-dialysis not widely available.
Oral phosphate binders	Calcium-containing: calcium carbonate calcium acetate	Hypercalcaemia Increase total body calcium Evidence of progressive vascular calcification	Used widely Useful in hypocalcaemia
	Aluminium hydroxide	Osteomalacia, adynamic bone disease, microcytic anaemia 'Dialysis dementia'	Very effective and inexpensive K/DOQI guidelines restrict usage to high calcium-phosphate product and duration of treatment to 4 weeks
	Non-calcium, non-aluminium containing: Sevelamer, Lanthanum	Abdominal pain Metabolic acidosis	Relatively expensive Ameliorate progression of vascular calcification in haemodialysis patients
Vitamin D analogues	Calcitriol 1-alfa-calcidol, Paricalcitol	Hypercalcaemia and hyper-phosphataemia	Over-suppression of PTH may cause adynamic bone disease
Parathyroidectomy	Total or 3/4 parathyroid-ectomy	Surgical risk Hypocalcaemia may ensue	Very effective treatment of otherwise refractory secondary hyperpara-thyroidism

Figure 6.6 Treatment of secondary hyperparathyroidism in CKD

Therapy	Drugs	Side effects	Comments
Calcimimetics	Cinacalcet	Vomiting at beginning of treatment Hypocalcaemia	Daily treatment and potentially life-long (therefore expensive compared to parathyroid-ectomy). Reduces incidence of parathyroidectomy in patients with secondary hyperparathyroidism
Injection of parathyroid nodules	Absolute alcohol, Calcitriol		Little expertise in UK

Figure 6.6 cont. Treatment of secondary hyperparathyroidism in CKD

New drugs are currently being introduced to clinical practice that increase CaSR sensitivity to extracellular ionised calcium, thereby inhibiting the release of PTH. These drugs are referred to as calcimimetics and cinacalcet hydrochloride is the first in class that has been tested in randomised trials. In the UK, NICE have recommended that use of cinacalcet should be restricted to patients with refractory (tertiary) hyperparathyroidism if surgical parathyroidectomy is contraindicated. Currently, to qualify for this treatment, plasma concentrations of PTH must exceed 800 ng/L (84.8 pmol/L). Given the increasing recognition that abnormalities in calcium and phosphate homeostasis contribute to cardiovascular risk in CKD, such drugs may have a greater role in the future.

Anaemia

Definitions
The World Health Organisation defines anaemia as a haemoglobin concentration of < 12 g/dL in women and < 13 g/dL in men. The NKF K/DOQI defines anaemia in CKD as a haemoglobin concentration of < 11 g/dL in pre-menopausal females and pre-pubertal patients, and < 12 g/dL in adult males and post-menopausal females. The Revised European Best Practice Guidelines (EBPG) define anaemia as a haemoglobin concentration two standard deviations below the population mean, i.e. < 11.5 g/dL in adult female patients, < 13.5 g/dL in adult male patients, and < 12.0 g/dL in adult male patients aged > 70 years. The UK Renal Association Standards recommend evaluation of anaemia 'when haemoglobin < 13 g/dL (adult males and post-menopausal females), < 12 g/dL (pre-menopausal females)' and that 'anaemia is more likely to be the result of CKD if the GFR is < 30 mL/min/1.73 m^2 (< 45 mL/min/1.73 m^2 in diabetics) and no other cause, e.g. blood loss, folate or B$_{12}$ deficiency, is identified'.

In the absence of treatment, anaemia is universal in ESRD patients. Prior to the introduction of erythropoiesis-stimulating agents (ESAs) in the 1980s, most dialysis patients had haemoglobin concentrations < 10 g/dL and often much lower. Detection of anaemia is important since, if left untreated, it causes many of the side effects of CKD such as fatigue, breathlessness on exertion, intolerance to cold and decreased exercise capacity. Anaemia is also associated with development of cardiovascular disease in patients with CKD, in particular LVH.

Pathobiology of renal anaemia
The aetiology of anaemia in CKD is multi-factorial and it is well established that anaemia is inevitable as CKD progresses. Data from Canada have shown that anaemia is present in around 25% of patients with CKD whose GFR is > 50 mL/min, 44% between 35-49 mL/min, 51% between 25-34 mL/min, and 87% below 25 mL/min. Data from the third NHANES study suggest that the decline in haemoglobin concentration starts at a GFR of 70 mL/min in men and 50 mL/min in women.

A major cause of anaemia is the loss of peritubular fibroblasts within the renal cortex that synthesise EPO. EPO is a large glycoprotein hormone (Mr 34 kDa) containing 165 amino acids and is responsible for stimulating erythroid progenitor cells within the bone marrow to produce red blood cells. Failure of EPO production in the kidney leads to inappropriately low concentrations within the blood for the concomitant concentration of haemoglobin. Other causes of anaemia include absolute or functional iron deficiency, folic acid and vitamin B_{12} deficiencies, and chronic inflammation. Red cell survival may also be reduced. Haemodialysis patients tend to have more severe anaemia than peritoneal dialysis patients because of greater blood losses during dialysis.

Investigation of renal anaemia
Therapies are available to correct anaemia and therefore it is mandatory to assess a patient with CKD for anaemia. Assessment involves establishing the contribution of iron deficiency and, initially, excluding vitamin B_{12} and folate deficiencies. Serum ferritin measurement is used to assess iron stores, whereas measurement of transferrin saturation gives an indication of iron 'delivery'. Patients with CKD stage 5 can be diagnosed as being iron deficient when the serum ferritin concentration is < 100 µg/L. In stage 3 and 4 CKD, iron deficiency anaemia can be *considered* when the serum ferritin concentration is < 100 µg/L. 'Functional' iron deficiency is defined by serum ferritin concentration > 100 µg/L and either a transferrin saturation of < 20% or percentage of hypochromic red blood cells > 6%. Limitations with these indices exist: a high ferritin concentration may also be secondary to an inflammatory process and transferrin concentration varies with nutritional state and is also influenced by inflammation.

Management of renal anaemia

The recently published guidelines from NICE in England and Wales provide a valuable resource for the management of anaemia in people with CKD. The key priorities for implementation of the guidelines include management of anaemia in adult patients with CKD when the haemoglobin is less than or equal to 11 g/dL. Treatment should be aimed at maintaining a stable haemoglobin of 10.5-12.5 g/dL in adults.

Treatment of anaemia in CKD requires adequate iron stores and, where appropriate, introduction of ESAs. Iron correction should maintain serum ferritin concentration > 200 µg/L, transferrin saturation > 20% and, where the test is available, hypochromic red blood cells < 6%. Parenteral iron is often used since oral iron has low efficacy in CKD, particularly among haemodialysis patients. The UK Renal Association recommends regular monitoring (1-3 monthly) of iron status in patients receiving replacement treatment; a serum ferritin concentration > 800 µg/L may suggest iron overload.

Following optimisation of iron status, treatment with ESAs should be offered to people with anaemia and CKD who are likely to benefit in terms of quality of life and function. ESAs are recombinant erythropoietins; currently available ESAs include epoetin alfa, epoetin beta, darbepoetin alfa and methoxy polyethylene-glycol epoetin beta. ESAs are inactive when given by mouth and must therefore be given parenterally, either intravenously or subcutaneously. Intravenous administration is practical for some haemodialysis patients. ESA treatment is effective at correcting the anaemia of CKD in 90-95% of patients. The UK Renal Association recommends monitoring of haemoglobin concentration at least 1-3 monthly in dialysis patients receiving ESAs, with dosage adjustment accordingly. The most common side effect is hypertension, which may develop or worsen in a quarter of patients. Blood pressure should therefore be well controlled prior to the introduction of treatment. Measurement of serum EPO concentration is rarely indicated in the setting of renal anaemia.

It is estimated that at least 3 million patients worldwide have received treatment with ESAs. There are many clinical benefits of correcting anaemia with ESA therapy, including improved exercise capacity, improved cognitive function, better quality of life, and increased libido. In advanced CKD, studies have suggested that regression of LVH is possible with partial correction of anaemia with ESAs. Clinical trials are ongoing to try to answer the key question as to whether early normalisation of anaemia in CKD will translate into improved cardiovascular outcomes. Patient education is a central component of anaemia management in CKD and ESAs may be self-administered by subcutaneous injection once to three times weekly. Long-acting ESAs e.g methoxy polyethylene-glycol epoetin beta, allow for depot dosing. Treatment plans are coordinated from the renal unit, with shared care protocols established between primary care and secondary care. Failure to respond to ESAs ('resistance', defined either as failure to reach the target haemoglobin concentration or the requirement for excessive dosages of ESAs) requires thorough investigation for many potential causes (Figure 6.7).

Failure to respond to erythropoiesis stimulating agents

Iron deficiency (absolute or functional) - commonest cause

Poor compliance with treatment

Occult blood loss

Vitamin B_{12} or folate deficiency

Infection or inflammation

Inadequate dialysis

Hyperparathyroidism

Aluminium toxicity

Hypothyroidism

Primary disease activity

Transplant rejection

Malignancy

Pure red cell aplasia

Figure 6.7 Failure to respond to erythropoiesis stimuating agents (ESAs)

Malnutrition

Deterioration in nutritional status often begins early in the course of CKD, particularly when the GFR falls below 30 mL/min/1.73 m^2. As a result, protein-energy malnutrition is frequently present at the time an individual commences dialysis. Malnutrition in patients commencing RRT is a strong predictor of poor clinical outcome. Dialysis patients tend to have a poor appetite, which may be exacerbated by depression or heart failure. Protein metabolism is also altered in the setting of chronic acidosis and low-grade inflammation or infection.

Nutritional screening is recommended in dialysis patients. Such screening may involve subjective global assessment (SGA), measurement of body mass index (BMI), eliciting a recent history of (oedema-free) weight loss, dietary history, measurement of serum albumin concentration and more recently, bioimpedance variables. The Renal Association has recommended that a diagnosis of undernutrition should be considered if any of the criteria listed in Figure 6.8 are satisfied.

Identifying undernutrition

A diagnosis of undernutrition should be considered if any of the following criteria are met:

• BMI < 18.5 kg/m^2

• Unintentional loss of oedema-free weight > 10% in past 6 months

• Low subjective global assessment score

Figure 6.8 Identifying undernutrition. (Adapted from the UK Renal Association Standards for Treatment of Adults and Children with Renal Failure, 3rd Edition, 2002).

Assessment of body composition is commonly included in the general examination of nutritional status. The SGA provides a score obtained from subjective and objective aspects of the medical history and physical examination that allows patients to be categorised as having either normal, mild, moderate or severe malnutrition. In patients with kidney disease, the presence of oedema may lead to an overestimate of the BMI; oedema-free weight should be assessed where possible. Single-frequency bioimpedance analysis can be utilised as a simple bedside or clinic technique. Derived values for fat-free mass and total body water can be estimated using predictive formulae that include bioimpedance variables.

Recently, it has been demonstrated that, in the absence of overt malnutrition, altered bioimpedance variables are exhibited early in CKD. These alterations are more marked in diabetes and mainly indicate the presence of over-hydration in the absence of oedema.

Despite its many limitations, serum albumin concentration is widely used as a marker of nutritional status in dialysis patients. Problems associated with the use of albumin as a marker of nutrition include the fact that hypoalbuminaemia is also associated with the acute-phase response, with concomitant increases of inflammatory markers, including C-reactive protein (CRP). Persistent elevation of CRP is common in dialysis patients, and may occur in the absence of detectable infection. Peritonitis may occur in patients treated by peritoneal dialysis (PD) and this causes significant albumin loss due to peritoneal membrane leakage. An additional difficulty is the variation in assays used, with bromocresol green (BCG) methods generally giving serum albumin results approximately 5 g/L higher than bromocresol purple (BCP) methods in the dialysis population. Not all BCG methods are equivalent, with the relative interference from non-albumin protein being in part dependent on the time period over which the reaction is monitored (non-albumin proteins react more slowly than albumin itself). Further, dry-slide BCG methods have in fact been reported to show a slight negative bias (-1 g/L) when compared to immunological assays. Although some authors have demonstrated improved accuracy of BCP methods compared to BCG in uraemic patients, others have shown significant underestimation of serum albumin by BCP methods in haemodialysis patients. This may relate to the presence of an inhibitor of the BCP dye-binding reaction that accumulates in haemodialysis patients but not in patients being treated with PD.

Reduction of body weight below reference values correlates with loss of body protein, as well as increased risk of hospitalisation, post-operative complications, and mortality. The recommended protein dietary requirements change as CKD progresses. In the pre-dialysis setting, daily protein intake is recommended at 0.8-1.0 g/kg ideal body weight. Increased requirements are recommended in patients receiving dialysis. In particular, patients treated by PD are encouraged to ingest 1.2-1.5 g/kg protein per day to compensate for protein losses across the peritoneal membrane. Calorie and protein supplements are offered to many patients with advanced CKD and those on RRT. Patients with stages 4 and 5 CKD and those receiving RRT have ready access to specialist renal dietitians for advice and supervision in most cases. In patients with a persistently high CRP, a source of infection should be sought and, where found, treated. Other catabolic factors such as acidosis, thyrotoxicosis and poor diabetic control should also be managed.

Hyperkalaemia

Although disturbances of plasma sodium and potassium concentration are caused by alterations in handling of water, sodium, and potassium in the kidney, these are frequently due to external influences (e.g. endocrine, drugs) on kidney function rather than primary disorders of the kidney. In these situations, the treatment is that of the underlying disorder. Referral to a nephrologist is reasonable when no cause is evident, because of the potentially serious consequences of each of these electrolyte abnormalities.

In health, approximately 90% of potassium loss occurs via renal excretion (see Chapter 1). Patients with kidney disease have impaired renal excretion of potassium. Hyperkalaemia, defined as a serum potassium concentration in excess of 5.5 mmol/L (approximately equivalent to a *plasma* potassium concentration of 5.0 mmol/L), is the electrolyte abnormality that occurs most frequently in CKD. Kidney disease is the most common cause of hyperkalaemia in patients presenting to hospital. It is of significance because severe hyperkalaemia (e.g. > 6.5 mmol/L) is associated with cardiac arrhythmias and can cause cardiac arrest and death with very few warning symptoms. Measurement of serum potassium concentration is recommended at least annually in patients with stage 3 CKD. In stage 4-5 CKD, hyperkalaemia becomes increasingly common as GFR declines, and may be an indication for starting RRT.

Some types of CKD, particularly diabetic nephropathy and interstitial nephritis, can be associated with suppression of renin and aldosterone release, causing hyperkalaemia disproportionate to the reduction in GFR. Drug treatment with ACE inhibitors and ARBs can contribute to hyperkalaemia, which can also be exacerbated by treatment with spironolactone (indicated in the treatment of heart failure), beta-blockers, and NSAIDs. Severe effective hypovolaemia, which may complicate the treatment of heart failure with high dose diuretics, may also cause hyperkalaemia in the presence of CKD. In the presence of volume overload diuretics however, may be a logical *treatment* for hyperkalaemia. For these reasons, working out the cause and appropriate treatment of hyperkalaemia can be difficult, and referral to a nephrologist is recommended. It must of course always be borne in mind that significant changes in potassium concentration can occur *in vitro* after venesection due to delay in laboratory processing or haemolysis. These problems may be exacerbated in the presence of thrombocytosis (high blood platelet count) or leucocytosis.

The UK Renal Association has recommended that predialysis serum potassium concentration should be between 3.5 and 6.5 mmol/L in HD patients. This is achieved through dietary restriction (particularly certain vegetables and fruits,

Figure 6.9) and avoidance of drugs that might contribute to hyperkalaemia (e.g. ACE inhibitors). A particular problem in this respect is the use of LoSalt®, a salt substitute that contains potassium chloride and which may be mistakenly ingested by ESRD patients. Dialysis itself is the major mechanism for removing potassium in ESRD patients and this can be facilitated with the use of low potassium dialysates. However, there is a danger of severe hypokalaemia postdialysis, which increases the risk of cardiac arrhythmias. The management of hyperkalaemia in the setting of ARF is discussed in Chapter 4.

Foods containing high concentrations of potassium
Fruits: bananas, dried fruit, rhubarb, avocados
Vegetables: mushrooms, potatoes, beans
Drinks: fruit juices, Bovril, coffee, cocoa, milk, beer
Others: LoSalt®, chocolate, potato crisps

Figure 6.9 Foods containing high concentrations of potassium.

Further reading

CARDIOVASCULAR DISEASE

Giachelli CM. Vascular calcification mechanisms. J Am Soc Nephrol 2004; **15:** 2959-64.

London G. Pathophysiology of cardiovascular damage in the early renal population. Nephrol Dial Transplant 2001; **16(suppl 2):** 3-6.

RENAL OSTEODYSTROPHY

Eknoyan G, Levin A, Levin NW. Bone metabolism and disease in chronic kidney disease. Am J Kidney Dis 2003; **42(suppl. 3):** 1-201.

ANAEMIA

National Institute of Health and Clinical Excellence (NICE). Anaemia management in people with chronic kidney disease at www.nice.org.uk/CG039. Issue date: September 2006.

National Kidney Foundation. KDOQI Clinical Practice Guidelines and Clinical Practice Recommendations for Anemia in Chronic Kidney Disease. Am J Kidney Dis 2006; **47 (suppl 3):** S1-S146.

Chapter 7

Renal replacement therapy

Background

In 1861, Thomas Graham Bell in Glasgow, Scotland carried out the first dialysis experiments (and coined the term 'dialysis'), separating crystalloids and colloids in a solution. Bell predicted that this technique could have a medical application. In 1913, Abel and his colleagues successfully removed salicylate from dogs by using a device to circulate blood through collodion tubes surrounded by a jacket filled with normal saline. It was not until 1944 that Willem Kolff introduced the first practical artificial kidney. The availability of dialysis was shown dramatically to reduce mortality from traumatic ARF during the Korean War in 1952. In 1960, Belding Scribner perfected the 'Scribner Shunt' utilising cannulae inserted into a suitable peripheral artery and one into a suitable vein. The cannulae were connected with a rigid piece of Teflon over a stainless steel arm plate. This semi-permanent exteriorised arteriovenous shunt made repeated access to a patient's circulation possible. Cimino and Brescia described the formation of a subcutaneous arterio-venous fistula (AVF) between the radial artery and an adjacent vein in 1966, and this has remained the preferred mode of access to a patient's circulation for haemodialysis to this day (Figure 7.1).

Commencing renal replacement therapy

The timing of initiation of dialysis treatment is controversial. In symptomatic patients and those with severe metabolic derangements, it is generally obvious that RRT is required (Figure 7.2). There is debate as to whether early initiation of dialysis improves outcomes over late starters. The KDOQI 2006 Updates Clinical Practice Guidelines and Clinical Practice Recommendations suggest that the benefits, risks and disadvantages of beginning RRT should be evaluated by the physician on a case-by-case basis when the GFR falls below 15 mL/min/1.73 m². The mean estimated GFR in 2003 at initiation of dialysis therapy in the US was 9.8 mL/min/1.73 m², and approximately 8 mL/min/1.73 m² in the UK. Observational studies and registry data suggest that patients with diabetes and cardiovascular comorbid illness commence RRT at higher levels of GFR. Patients that reach Stage 4 CKD with evidence of progressive decline should receive education about kidney failure and available options for treatment. For selected patients, conservative therapy, without dialysis or transplantation, is the appropriate option. It has been acknowledged by the KDOQI Work Group that the initiation of dialysis therapy remains a decision that is informed by clinical art as well as science.

An arterio-venous fistula in a chronic haemodialysis patient

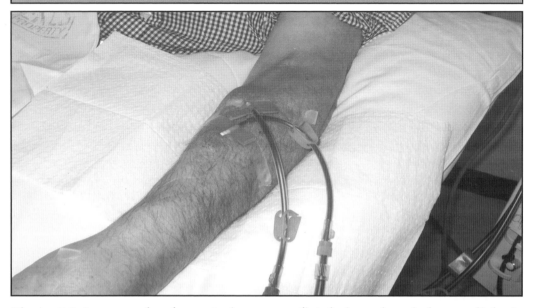

Figure 7.1 An example of an arterio-venous fistula in a chronic haemodialysis patient. The dialysis needles are placed in the arterialised vein with the arterial needle (right port) pointing towards the blood flow and the return ('venous' port just showing at bottom of picture) needle placed upstream and directed centrally to reduce recirculation of dialysed blood. This improves the clearance during a dialysis session.

Indications for initiating RRT

Hyperkalaemia refractory to medical treatment

Severe metabolic acidosis refractory to bicarbonate supplements

Uraemia (encephalopathy, pericarditis, bleeding)

Pulmonary oedema

Malnutrition and failure to thrive

GFR estimation confirming ESRD

Figure 7.2 Indications for initiating RRT

Haemodialysis and haemofiltration

Haemodialysis

Haemodialysis (HD) can be regarded as the default therapy that is utilised in the increasing numbers of patients unsuitable for other modalities of RRT e.g. peritoneal dialysis (PD) and kidney transplantation. HD is a technique used to remove toxic substances from the blood when the kidneys cannot satisfactorily remove them from the circulation. HD utilises diffusive and convective mass transfer across a semi-permeable membrane. The driving force for diffusion is the concentration gradient between blood and dialysate (dialysis fluid). Smaller solutes with larger concentration gradients diffuse more rapidly. To maintain a steep concentration gradient, heparinised blood is pumped in one direction across the membrane and the dialysate flows at a rate of 500-800 mL/min in the opposite direction. Dialysate is generated from a mixture of water, dialysis fluid electrolyte concentrate and bicarbonate. The composition of the dialysate is designed to resemble plasma water and is controlled by a proportioning system, which also acts to control concentration (conductivity) and temperature to pre-set limits.

Water and low molecular weight molecules can cross the dialyser membrane, while larger proteins and cellular elements are retained in the vascular space. Since convection is the bulk movement of solvent and dissolved solute across the membrane down a transmembrane hydrostatic pressure gradient, water transport is accomplished through creation of a pressure difference across the membrane (the transmembrane pressure). The ease with which solute is dragged across a membrane is described by its sieving coefficient: the ratio of its concentration in ultrafiltrate to its concentration in plasma. Conventional HD uses low ultrafiltration (UF) coefficient dialysers, allowing diffusive, but little convective solute removal. In this setting, middle molecule clearance is poor. These dialysers are termed 'low-flux'. In contrast, haemofiltration (HF) is a convective treatment. Although middle molecule clearances are improved, small molecule clearance is poor (Figure 7.3). HF is used for continuous treatment in intensive care units in the management of ARF.

The major components of the dialysis system include the patient, circulatory access, connecting lines to the artificial kidney (dialyser), and a dialysate delivery system. The outline of a typical haemodialyser circuit is shown in Figure 7.4. Dialysers are semi-permeable membranes classified by membrane composition, surface area, permeability characteristics and biocompatibility. Biocompatibility reflects the degree of inflammation that may occur during blood-membrane contact. A variety of membranes are available with different surface areas and filtration characteristics. The oldest type of membrane was made from cuprophane and cellulose acetate. However, these have been replaced by more biocompatible synthetic membranes made from polysulfone and polyacrylonitrile. Biocompatible membranes are more rigid (allowing higher flow rates) and have higher clearances of larger molecules such as β_2-microglobulin. Conflicting results have been obtained from studies looking at mortality and type of dialysis membrane used. The Cochrane Database of Systematic Reviews did not find evidence of benefit when synthetic membranes were compared with cellulose or modified-cellulose membranes with regard to mortality and dialysis-related adverse effects. This recent finding is at odds with modern clinical practice since the majority of UK renal units have converted their entire haemodialysis programme to the more biocompatible synthetic dialysers.

Molecular size and clearance in haemodialysis

Type of solute	Molecular weight (Daltons)	Mode of solute clearance
Small solutes (e.g. urea, creatinine, electrolytes, bicarbonate, phosphate)	< 300	Diffusion
Middle molecules (e.g. vitamin B_{12}, β_2-microglobulin, parathyroid hormone, cystatin C, vancomycin)	300 -12,000	Diffusion and convection
Large molecules (e.g. tumour necrosis factor, interleukins)	12,000-50,000	Convection and adsorption

Figure 7.3 Molecular size and clearance in haemodialysis

Dialysers are either hollow-fibre in structure or flat plate. Hollow-fibre dialysers contain bundles of thousands of fibres similar in structure to capillaries. By altering the applied pressure across the membrane, fluid removal by UF can be regulated, and by altering the flow rate of dialysate and blood, solute removal can be regulated. The main purpose of UF in dialysis is the therapeutic removal of fluid to treat fluid overload and to make room for eating and drinking prior to the next dialysis treatment.

The use of more porous membranes and 'high-flux' biocompatible membranes in HD allows increased convective and diffusive solute removal. The use of very pure water is crucial in high-flux modes because dialysis fluid is infused directly into the bloodstream by back filtration. The Hemodialysis (HEMO) Study, a National Institutes of Health-sponsored randomised clinical trial from the US, was designed to determine whether increasing the dose of dialysis or using a high-flux dialyser membrane rather than a low-flux dialyser membrane alters major clinical outcomes (mortality and hospitalisations). The HEMO Study Group concluded in 2002 that patients undergoing HD three times per week had no major benefit from a higher dialysis dose than that recommended by current guidelines or from the use of a high-flux membrane over a conventional low-flux membrane.

Schematic outline of a haemodialysis circuit

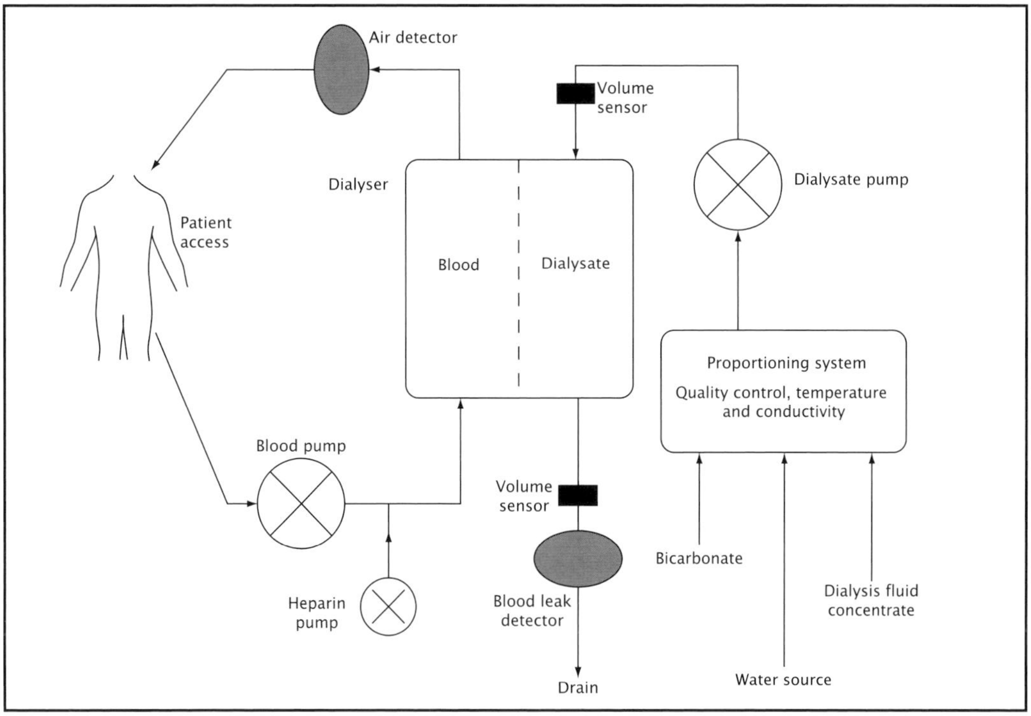

Figure 7.4 Schematic outline of a haemodialysis circuit. The addition of ultra-pure substitution fluid before or after the dialyser converts the circuit to haemodiafiltration.

Patients can be dialysed in home-based or hospital-based units, with dialysis usually performed three times a week for sessions lasting for between 3-5 hours. This dialysis schedule is largely empirical in so far as it reconciles adequate treatment with breaks between treatments to provide the patient with a reasonable quality of life. Approaches to increasing the dose of dialysis have been explored. These include short daily HD that entails 2-3 hours of dialysis on six days per week. Alternatively, slow overnight dialysis for 5-7 nights has been employed. These regimens are reported to improve outcome.

Haemofiltration

Haemofiltration is a convection-based blood cleansing technique. As blood flows through the filter, the transmembrane pressure gradient between the blood compartment and the ultrafiltrate department causes plasma water to be filtered across the membrane along with convection of small and large molecules. The ultrafiltrate is replaced by a balanced electrolyte solution infused at either the inflow or outflow line of the filter. This technique is commonly used in intensive care units to treat patients with ARF (Chapter 4). Intermittent haemofiltration has been used in place of intermittent haemodialysis. Using highly permeable haemofilters, 25-30 L of ultrafiltrate are removed per session, with infusion of the appropriate amount of sterile replacement fluid. Although there is a theoretical advantage of haemofiltration over haemodialysis in terms of removal of larger molecular weight putative uraemic toxins, this has not been demonstrated prospectively. The requirement for large volumes of sterile replacement fluid, with increased cost, has limited the use of this technique for maintenance RRT. However, modern dialysis machines now incorporate on-line production and delivery of sterile replacement fluid.

Haemodiafiltration

Haemodiafiltration (HDF) combines the use of a high-flux dialyser membrane with large volume convection, in which fluid removal exceeds the desired weight loss, and maintenance of fluid balance by the infusion of a sterile pyrogen-free solution. This technique offers the advantages of both HD and haemofiltration in a single therapy. The replacement fluid, previously supplied in autoclaved bags, is now generated 'on-line' from concentrated bicarbonate and uses 20-30 L of water per session. The result is that HDF provides a 10-15% increase in urea clearance compared with HD and markedly increased middle molecule clearances. Water for on-line preparation of substitution solution should meet common standards for dialysis water regarding chemical contaminants, but have a higher quality regarding microbiological contaminants. It should be free from bacteria and pyrogens (i.e. ultrapure). Dialysis water is purified using a combination of techniques including softening and deionisation, carbon adsorption, dual-pass reverse osmosis and ultraviolet irradiation. On-line HDF has been used extensively in continental Europe over the past 15 years or so, and there is evidence that long-term complications of dialysis, such as carpal tunnel syndrome, may be reduced. The hypothesis is that increased clearance of middle molecules, such as β_2-microglobulin in the blood, helps to reduce accumulation of these proteins. Several trials have found a measurable effect of high-flux dialysis and HDF on the concentration of β_2-microglobulin. However, a recent Cochrane Database Systematic Review was unable to demonstrate whether or not convective modalities (either HF or HDF) have significant advantages over HD in terms of mortality and cardiovascular morbidity.

The modality of extra-corporeal blood cleansing treatment chosen in the chronic population is generally limited to either conventional haemodialysis or to haemodiafiltration. There are increased costs associated with HDF over HD and this may limit the use of HDF in some centres. On occasions, patients that remain unstable on HD despite measures to maintain intra-dialytic blood pressure may be treated with a trial of HDF. In centres where HDF is not universal, individual selection criteria may be considered. For example, a young patient that is unlikely to receive a kidney transplant and who will therefore require dialysis for many years, may benefit from HDF instead of HD to reduce complications of dialysis-related amyloid.

Fluid management

Fluid management on HD is crucial to patient well being and survival. Since conventional dialysis is based on a three times per week schedule, fluid is accumulated by the patient between dialysis sessions. Many patients are anuric or at least oliguric and therefore unrestricted fluid intake would result in fluid overload and complications of pulmonary oedema and hypertension. Patients receiving HD are advised to restrict fluid intake to 1 L/24 h or so. This allowance is recommended to the individual patient by the dialysis nursing staff and dietician to ensure adequate nutrition is maintained. Nevertheless, many patients find the fluid restriction very difficult to maintain and therefore large weight gains between dialysis sessions are a common occurrence. During the dialysis session, the patient's 'dry' or 'target' weight is achieved. The dry weight assumes that the fluid compartments are normal and is determined by gradually reducing weight until the patient is oedema-free but before hypotension occurs. This is difficult to reach in patients with abnormal cardiovascular responses who may become hypotensive despite being relatively fluid replete.

When haemodialysis therapy is first initiated, most patients have a small amount of residual renal function (RRF). This level of RRF may persist for many months and years and the volume of urine produced each day allows more fluid intake, but also has the benefit of reducing large fluctuations in body fluid volumes. RRF should be taken into consideration when adjusting dialysis prescriptions. The KDOQI Work Group 2006 Updates include recommendations, as opposed to guidelines (opinion-based rather than evidence-based), for preserving RRF in patients receiving HD (Figure 7.5).

Assessing dialysis adequacy in haemodialysis

The assessment of adequacy of dialysis treatment for individual patients in the clinical setting includes consideration of the patient's well being, cardiovascular risk, nutritional status, degree of achievable UF, laboratory estimates of a number of parameters such as haemoglobin, phosphate and albumin, and clearance of the small solutes urea and creatinine. During the following discussion, the term 'adequacy' will refer to small solute clearances obtained from both dialysis and RRF. For practical reasons, HD adequacy is calculated using urea as the small solute. The overall clearance of a solute by dialysis is equal to the sum of its diffusive and convective clearance. For any given dialyser this will depend on blood and dialysate flow rates, the UF rate, and the concentrations of solute in blood and dialysate. Urea kinetic modelling (UKM) is used to assess adequacy. The kinetics of urea removal during dialysis and the inter-dialytic regeneration of urea between sessions are modelled using computer software to calculate the clearance of urea during that dialysis session and is expressed as the index Kt/V_{urea}. This index is now the most commonly used assessment of the adequacy of haemodialysis, where K is the effective urea clearance in mL/min integrated over the entire dialysis, t is the time in minutes measured from the beginning to the end of dialysis and V is the patient's volume of distribution of urea in mL. The only measurements required are pre- and post-dialysis urea, duration of dialysis and weight loss during dialysis.

Strategies to preserve renal function in dialysis patients

- Avoidance of nephrotoxic agents (especially aminoglycosides, NSAIDs, cyclooxygenase-2 inhibitors and radiocontrast media)

- Avoidance of excessive ultrafiltration and intra-dialytic hypotension

- Routine use of biocompatible dialyser membrane

- Aggressive treatment of hypertension

- Use of ACE inhibitors and/or ARBs

- Use of ultrapure dialysate

Figure 7.5 Strategies to preserve renal function in dialysis patients

In practice, rather than using full UKM, a more straightforward calculation is the urea reduction ratio (URR). The percentage fall in serum urea attained during a dialysis session is measured as follows:

$$\frac{\text{Pre-dialysis [urea]} - \text{post-dialysis [urea]}}{\text{Pre-dialysis urea}} \quad X\ 100\%$$

The URR does not take convective removal of urea or RRF into account. Its accuracy is lower than Kt/V measured by formal UKM, particularly at high values of URR and Kt/V. The target URR is 70% in patients who receive dialysis three times each week. In general, the minimum standard for thrice weekly haemodialysis is a Kt/V of 1.2 per dialysis. The Kt/V effectively describes the *power* of the dialysis session. A retrospective analysis of the National Cooperative Dialysis Study was the first to identify a threshold in level of Kt/V and outcomes in HD. Data from the HEMO study revealed a coefficient of variation within patients of approximately 0.1 Kt/V units, therefore the recently published recommendations from the KDOQI Work Group in the US and the European Standards Group is a *target* Kt/V of at least 1.4 per dialysis.

Peritoneal dialysis

Background
Peritoneal dialysis (PD) was first explored by Ganter in 1923 and initially showed poor results. The modern era only really started in 1953, with intermittent irrigation of the peritoneal cavity with commercially prepared solutions and access achieved through a single disposable catheter. Popovich and co-workers in 1976 introduced the concept of portable equipment and this approach developed into continuous ambulatory peritoneal dialysis (CAPD). This form of dialysis is now widely used across the world. The percentage of incident and prevalent patients receiving PD has declined in the US over recent years, particularly in older people. Between 8-10% of dialysis patients were treated with PD in the US in 2002, with HD remaining the default treatment modality for RRT. Uptake of PD varies between countries depending on access to haemodialysis. For example, in the UK, 31% of prevalent patients receive PD and in Mexico 90% of patients receive PD.

Principles of PD
PD utilises the patient's own peritoneal membrane (surface area approximately 2 m^2) across which fluid and solutes can be exchanged between the peritoneal capillary blood and the dialysis solution placed in the peritoneal cavity (Figure 7.6). A catheter (Tenchkoff catheter) is inserted below the umbilicus into the abdominal cavity and then tunnelled subcutaneously to a lateral exit site. The catheter is connected via lines to bags of PD fluid. After an exchange (draining effluent out and running a new clear bag in), the lines are disconnected and the patient remains independent until the next exchange several hours later. Fluid removal or UF is achieved by using dialysis fluids containing a high concentra-

tion of glucose which acts as an osmotic agent. The PD fluid bags have differing concentrations of glucose in them (76, 126 and 214 mmol/L), with the highest concentrations having the greatest osmotic effect (i.e. are the strongest bags for drawing fluid into the peritoneal space and increasing UF). As glucose passes across the peritoneal membrane, the rate of fluid removal decreases since the osmotic load of the peritoneal fluid is reduced.

Diagrammatic sketch of peritoneal dialysis

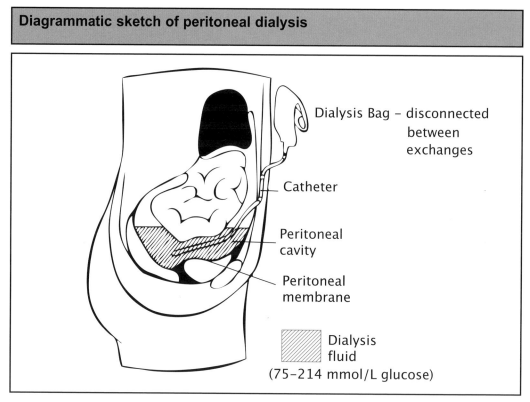

Figure 7.6 Diagrammatic sketch of peritoneal dialysis.

Conventional therapies use four exchanges of approximately 2 L of fluid resulting in the generation of approximately 10 L of spent dialysate (including UF) during a 24 hour period. This is repeated daily. The RRF is generally considered critical to the success of PD, since only a few mL/min can contribute substantially to urea and creatinine clearance, with each additional mL resulting in an extra 10 L of clearance per week. Positive reasons for opting for PD include preservation of RRF and vascular access sites and increased patient autonomy, since PD is performed by the patient in the home environment. Treatment can be administered at many locations and self-treatment is easier, with lower capital costs. The patient and relatives undergo a course of education and training delivered by specialist nurses, ensuring that the patient is motivated to achieve the maximum benefits of the treatment in the long-term. The higher permeability of the peritoneal membrane provides good removal of β_2-microglobulin and may help to protect patients on PD from the development of dialysis-related amyloid and carpal tunnel syndrome. Blood pressure control and extremes of fluid shifts are less problematic than with HD.

Glucose has been used as the osmotic agent in PD for 30 years, since the introduction of the technique. However, there are concerns over the amount of glucose that is absorbed and the effect of high glucose concentrations on protein glycation. The glucose solutions contribute calories and increase insulin requirements in patients with diabetes. Alternative, non-glucose osmotic agents have been developed. These include icodextrin, which is a solution of a starch-based glucose polymer, and amino acid based solutions. Since icodextrin is metabolised to maltose and other oligosaccharides following peritoneal absorption, false glucose readings may be obtained with some point-of-care blood monitoring systems. This is apparent where the glucose test uses a glucose dehydrogenase method. Systems that utilise a glucose oxidase reaction are safer for use in diabetic subjects receiving icodextrin (see box). Malnutrition is a potential complication of PD and is associated with increased morbidity and mortality. Loss of protein, which may amount to several g/day, and amino acids into the dialysate contribute to this problem. Several studies have shown that one exchange with a 1.1% amino acid dialysis solution is sufficient to compensate for losses and to improve nitrogen balance.

The manufacturer of icodextrin gives the following advice: since falsely elevated glucose levels have been observed with blood glucose monitoring devices and test strips that use glucose dehydrogenase pyrroloquinolinequinone (GDH PQQ) or glucose-dye-oxidoreductase-based methods, these methods should not be used to measure glucose levels in patients administered EXTRANEAL®. Falsely elevated glucose levels may mask true hypoglycemia or lead to the erroneous diagnosis of hyperglycaemia and administration of more insulin than needed. Both of these situations can result in loss of consciousness, coma, neurological damage and death. The manufacturer(s) of the monitor and test strips should be contacted to determine if icodextrin or maltose causes interference or falsely elevated glucose results.
www.baxter.com/products/renal/peritoneal_dialysis/sub/solutions.html. This problem has also been the subject of a Medicines and Healthcare products Regulatory Agency (MHRA) hazard notice (MDA/2003/011, obtainable at: www.mhra.gov.uk).

In addition to the manual exchanges that occur in CAPD, many units worldwide now offer a semi-automated delivery system for PD, so called 'automated PD' (APD). This requires a programmable machine to regulate dialysis fluid flow, intraperitoneal dwell time and drainage. It can be performed at night with the machine cycling the dialysis fluid in and out of the peritoneum at a pre-defined rate. This technique is a very convenient mode of dialysis. Solute clearance can be increased by leaving fluid in the peritoneum during the day and by performing an additional daytime exchange.

Assessment of adequacy in PD

A series of clinical outcome reports have demonstrated that measures of PD solute removal correlate to patient status and outcome. In particular, a multicentre prospective cohort study of 680 incident CAPD patients [Canada-United States (CANUSA) Study] showed that a decrease of 0.1 in weekly urea clearance (defined by Kt/V_{urea}) was associated with a 5% increase in the relative risk of death. Similarly, a decrease of 5 L/week/1.73 m^2 of total creatinine clearance (C_{Cr}) was associated with a 7% increase in the risk for death (Figure 7.7). As a consequence of these studies, national guidelines from the UK, Australia and USA have set standards of dialysis adequacy in terms of small solute removal.

Relative mortality risk for peritoneal dialysis patients		
Variable	**Relative risk**	
Age	1.03	for each year older
Diabetes	1.45	if present
Cardiovascular disease	2.09	if present
Kt/V	0.94	for each extra 0.1/week
Creatinine clearance	0.93	for each extra 5 L/week

Figure 7.7 Relative mortality risk for peritoneal dialysis patients (data taken from the CANUSA study, see Further reading)

An estimate of adequacy is performed in all patients within 6-8 weeks of commencement of PD. Further studies are performed at least annually. Defining adequacy in PD is confounded by the concern that solute removal by PD may not be clinically equivalent to solute removal by RRF. For PD, small-solute clearance targets have often been established on the assumption that peritoneal and renal clearances are equivalent and therefore additive. However, most studies that examined the relationship between small-solute clearances and mortality rates noted that patient survival was directly correlated with renal clearance. A recent prospective intervention trial from Mexico showed no additional benefit of increasing peritoneal clearance over the standard dialysis prescription in terms of mortality rates. Additionally, the value of assessing dialysis adequacy in terms of small solute removal has been questioned from the theoretical point of view, given that the relationship between these markers and the unidentified 'uraemic toxins' is not known. This is particularly pertinent to PD, given that it provides increased clearance of larger molecules compared to haemodialysis.

In the setting of PD, the elimination of two markers has typically been used to give an assessment of dialysis adequacy. Measurements of urea in both dialysate and blood are used to generate the parameter Kt/V. These, in combination with C_{Cr}, determined using measurements of creatinine in blood, dialysate and urine, are used to give an assessment of dialytic adequacy. To obtain the weekly Kt/V_{urea} requires the measurement of volume of spent dialysate and urine for a complete 24 h period. The concentration of urea in dialysate compared to plasma is calculated (the D/P ratio). This value is multiplied by the volume of the drained effluent to give an estimate of Kt. The calculation of 'V' or volume of distribution of urea is derived from an estimate of total body water. An estimate of weekly Kt/V_{urea} is simply the daily clearance multiplied by a factor of seven. These equations are used for both peritoneal and renal clearance and the total weekly clearance obtained by addition. Measurements of urea in plasma, urine and dialysis fluid also enable calculation of the normalised protein catabolic rate, a marker of protein intake in steady state conditions, which may have prognostic significance.

The calculation of C_{Cr} is based on the clearance (C) formula:

$$C = U \text{ (or D) } V/P$$

where U is the concentration of creatinine in urine or dialysate, V is the mean daily drain volume or urine volume (measured in litres) and P is the concentration of creatinine in the plasma.

Compliance with complete collections is mandatory. To avoid sampling errors, urine can be collected over 48 hours in those patients that void infrequently. The dialysate sampling requires all effluent bags in a 24 hour period to be brought to the centre renal unit. This can be difficult since the bags are heavy and bulky. In CAPD, plasma concentrations of urea and creatinine are relatively constant, and therefore blood can be drawn at any convenient time for clearance determinations. In APD, blood samples are typically collected after the overnight dialysis period. Both creatinine and urea concentrations can be obtained on the same sample of urine, blood and dialysate. It is important that glucose interference in the dialysate creatinine measurement is accounted for (e.g. by using an enzymatic creatinine method). The limitations of creatinine and creatinine clearance measurements have been discussed in Chapter 3, but in the setting of PD adequacy assessment, it should particularly be noted that it is especially compromised at low GFR, due to increased tubular secretion of creatinine and decreasing accuracy of the urine collection.

An adjunct to the assessment of adequacy in PD patients is the peritoneal equilibration test (PET), developed in Missouri, USA in the mid 1980s by Twardowski and colleagues to assess peritoneal membrane transport characteristics in terms of solute clearances and UF. Under controlled conditions, a dialysis exchange is performed and blood samples taken at 0 and 4 hours during the dwell period. After 4 hours, the dialysate is drained over 20 minutes and mixed well prior to aspirating a dialysate (D) sample. The blood and dialysate are analysed for creatinine and glucose. The UF can be calculated by weighing the clamped dialysis bag. In patients with high solute transport, the 4 hour glucose concentration is relatively low since the glucose in the dialysate is rapidly transported across the peritoneal membrane. The dialysate:plasma (D/P) creatinine ratio is calculated, with high values indicating rapid transfer of creatinine from blood to dialysate and high solute clearances. The membrane transport characteristics link solute clearances to UF, as the osmotic forces provided by glucose are lost during the dwell. Patients with very high or high-average transport characteristics show a rapid drop in dialysate glucose and a high D/P creatinine ratio. They usually have a diminished volume of UF due to rapid dissolution of the osmotic gradient between blood and dialysate across the peritoneal membrane. It is important to determine the membrane characteristics within 4-8 weeks after starting dialysis to obtain a baseline measurement. High transporter status patients benefit from short dwell times to maximise UF. Automated PD with short dwell times and programmable machines are utilised overnight to maintain solute clearance and adequate UF. In addition, icodextrin, the non-glucose osmotic agent, may be used to increase UF. Membrane function at the commencement of PD, measured as solute transport rate and UF capacity, varies considerably between individuals. It has been determined that high solute transport characteristics increase mortality risk independently of other known factors such as age, co-morbidity and RRF. In addition, fast transporters typically demonstrate evidence of systemic inflammation, although the underlying mechanisms have not been fully elucidated. In general peritoneal transport is stable over time. However, with increasing time on dialysis the amount of UF that can be achieved falls. Clinical indications for repeating a PET include unexplained volume overload, decreasing drain volume, increasing need for hypertonic dialysate dwells, worsening hypertension, uraemia symptoms and change in measured peritoneal solute removal. The UK Renal Association Standards document recommends at least annual assessment of peritoneal membrane transport kinetics. The PET is typically undertaken at the same time as adequacy assessments in PD patients. The measurement of adequacy is burdensome, labour intensive and prone to multiple measurement errors. Although dialysis centre nursing staff and patients may collect the necessary samples required for adequacy testing with the utmost diligence, the very complexity and number of measurements taken will cause systematic errors. Nevertheless, in the opinion of the authors of NKF-KDOQI Clinical Practice

Guidelines for PD Adequacy, these measures are reproducible enough to be useful in routine clinical practice. However, an alternative, simpler method for defining dialysis adequacy would be very useful in practice.

Peritonitis

One of the potential complications of PD is the development of peritoneal bacterial infection from contamination, leading to peritonitis. Incidence rates of peritonitis have decreased over the years with the introduction of disconnect PD systems, improved training of patients with regard to meticulous hygiene, and microbiological surveillance protocols. The current standard from the UK Renal Association is that the peritonitis rate should be less than one episode per 18 patient months. Peritonitis typically presents with a cloudy PD effluent and abdominal pain. Additional features, such as vomiting and a high temperature, suggest serious infection. Urgent samples must be taken for microbiological analysis and antibiotics administered via the PD tube directly into the peritoneum. If antibiotic treatment fails, the PD catheter is removed and the patient converted to HD. In the majority of cases, the episode of peritonitis responds to treatment and PD can continue, although it is likely that repeated episodes will cause scarring and fibrosis of the peritoneal membrane with permanent loss of UF. Long-term serious complications can occur, such as sclerosing encapsulating peritonitis caused by adhesions and peritoneal thickening encasing the peritoneal contents and causing bowel obstruction. This unusual condition is associated with increasing frequency of peritonitis episodes and longer duration of PD.

Kidney transplantation

Introduction

Joseph Murray, in Boston USA, performed the first successful kidney transplant in 1954 when he performed a donor transplant from one twin to the other. In 1959, Dameshek and Schwartz used 6-mercaptopurine (6-MP) in place of irradiation to precondition patients for bone marrow transplantation. Sir Roy Calne developed this work with the introduction of a safer derivative of 6-MP called azathioprine (AZT). By 1963, maintenance AZT and corticosteroids became the standard regimen for kidney transplantation. Kidney transplant or 'graft' survival with these treatment protocols was approximately 40% at 1 year. In the late 1970s and early 1980s ciclosporin was introduced. In combination with AZT and corticosteroids, it has been the mainstay immunosuppressive regimen. Ciclosporin based protocols led to fewer episodes of acute rejection and improved graft survival to 80-90% at 1 year. Tacrolimus was introduced during the 1990s and more recently mycophenolate mofetil (MMF) and sirolimus (Rapamycin) have been developed for use in kidney transplantation. Concurrently there has been marked progress with the use of biological agents (mono- or polyclonal antibodies directed against immune response cellular targets) to suppress the immune response to a graft in human transplant recipients. All these advances have led to increases in graft and patient survival, which are now in excess of 90% at 1 year. By contrast, long-term graft survival remains a major problem with half of transplants failing within 12 years, usually as a result of chronic allograft nephropathy (CAN) or death with a functioning graft. Recent data predict that the half-life will increase to almost 14 years for deceased donor (cadaveric donor) grafts.

The transplant waiting list

Kidney transplantation is the most effective form of RRT, in terms of long-term survival and quality of life. During the past 20 years, there have been more than 400,000 organ transplants performed in the US and there are currently 70,000 patients on the waiting list for a kidney transplant in the US alone. A further 2,395 are awaiting combined kidney and pancreas transplantation. There is a shortage of kidneys available for transplantation. In the UK, there has been a decline in the number of cadaveric donor transplants since 1992. Some of the shortfall has been addressed by increasing the supply of kidneys from live donation, with a 3-fold increase in the use of live donor transplants and no long-term detriment to the donor left with a single kidney. There is also evidence to suggest that the very best outcomes are achieved following pre-emptive live donor transplants (i.e. patients receive the transplant before undergoing dialysis treatment). Perioperative mortality for living kidney donors is reported at 0.03%. An alternative method for organ procurement is the use of nonheartbeating donors. Although only slowly accepted as feasible, recent data suggest good long-term outcomes. The waiting list for a kidney transplant reported by UK Transplant (UKT) in 2007 has reached almost 6,000 people in the UK, accounting for the majority of all patients awaiting an organ transplant (Figure 7.8).

Although patients with ESRD should have equitable access to kidney transplantation, currently only 23.3% of adult patients on dialysis are on the active renal transplant waiting list. The joint analyses between the UK Renal Registry and UK Transplant in England and Wales (2005) noted wide variations in practice between centres for listing patients for transplantation. In addition, time to transplant listing is dependent on age and primary renal disease. Older patients and those with renovascular disease are least likely to be listed, due to associated co-morbidity. The 23 year old age group has the highest proportion of patients on the active waiting list at 63% . In contrast, only 6-8% of 70 year old dialysis patients are on the active waiting list in England and Wales.

Waiting lists for all organ transplants 1997-2006

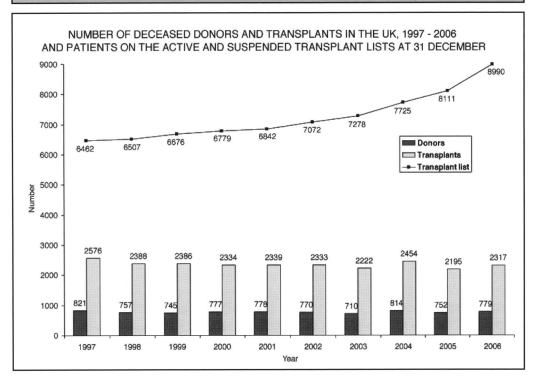

NUMBER OF DECEASED DONORS AND TRANSPLANTS IN THE UK, 1997 - 2006
AND PATIENTS ON THE ACTIVE AND SUSPENDED TRANSPLANT LISTS AT 31 DECEMBER

Figure 7.8 Cadaveric donor transplantation and the waiting list for all organ transplants, including kidney transplant waiting list 1997-2006.
Statistics prepared by UK Transplant from the National Transplant Database maintained on behalf of transplant services in the UK and Republic of Ireland. Patients on the suspended transplant list have been removed temporarily from the active list due to complicating clinical factors, but can be re-activated when circumstances allow. UK transplant statistics can be found at:
www.uktransplant.org.uk/ukt/statistics/statistics.jsp
UK Transplant is an operating division of NHS Blood and Transplant (NHSBT)

Waiting time spent on dialysis has been shown to be an important factor in determining mortality. In England and Wales, 45% of patients under the age of 65 years were placed on the transplant list within 1 year of starting dialysis and 66% within 5 years. The guideline published by UK Transplant is that people should be eligible for the national transplant list if dialysis is predicted to start within 6 months, typically with a GFR < 15 mL/min/1.73 m^2. The average time spent on the waiting list until transplantation is 841 days. The criteria for acceptance into a transplant program differ slightly from centre to centre, and the recent analysis by the joint UK Renal Registry and UK Transplant suggests this cannot be explained by either differences in patient case-mix or centre characteristics and is most likely to reflect a selection bias by healthcare professionals.

Increasing the number of donor kidneys is a major contemporary challenge. Recent evidence suggests that only 42% of potential deceased donors become actual donors in the US. Comparable figures have been recorded from the UK. Major initiatives have recently been introduced to increase the use of organs from potential donors. In the UK, two new acts came into force during 2006; the Human Tissue Act 2004 (covering England, Wales and Northern Ireland) and the Scottish equivalent, the Human Tissue (Scottish) Act 2006. The Acts place active consent at the centre. If the wishes of a potential donor are known concerning organ donation, they are paramount and cannot be overridden. A potential donor may register on the NHS Organ Donor Registry (www.uktransplant.org.uk). In practice, it is likely that organs will not be retrieved if the relatives of a potential donor object strongly to donation. In addition, the Acts regulate all aspects of living donation, make paired and altruistic non-directed donation lawful and allow *in situ* cold perfusion of organs after cardiac death without consent until such time as relatives are available to give or refuse permission for organ donation. It is anticipated that the deceased donor rate in the UK will increase above the current level of 12.8 per million population.

Transplant work-up of the recipient

Potential recipients must be screened to exclude those at high risk of perioperative mortality or premature death following transplantation. Preoperative assessment of a potential transplant recipient includes general health performance such as exercise capacity, general history and examination to identify co-morbidities such as diabetes and cardiovascular disease, and attention to the possibility of exclusion criteria that are suggested in Figure 7.9. Laboratory investigations are summarised in Figure 7.10. Further investigation depends on the individual patient and may include electrocardiogram, chest X-ray, two-dimensional transthoracic echocardiography and, in some cases, cardiac stress testing. Invasive investigation and treatment may be required. In addition, the potential recipient and relatives undergo counselling and education sessions.

Although a detailed description of the immunological aspects of transplantation is beyond the scope of this book, a brief discussion follows to highlight the close collaboration between clinicians and the tissue typing laboratory and to explore some of the recent advances in transplantation. The tissue type identifies an individual based on human leucocyte antigens (HLA) expressed on cells. These antigens are coded by genes of the major (and minor) histo- (tissue) compatibility complex (MHC). Individuals who have received blood transfusions, previous transplants of non-identical tissue, and females who have had pregnancies, develop antibodies to non-self HLA. These antibodies can be detected by analysing the recipient's serum against a panel of cells containing various HLA types. If there is a reaction between donor cells and recipient serum *in vitro* then this is indicative of a potential cross-reaction between donor organ and recipient at the time of transplantation. All recipients are tested regularly by the tissue typing service. Highly sensitive individuals have a number of antibodies or an antibody to a common HLA type and typically have a longer waiting time for a suitable donor kidney.

Exclusion criteria for consideration for a kidney transplant

Serious concomitant illness (particularly if likely to shorten life expectancy or be exacerbated by immunosuppressive treatment)

    Active malignancy*

    Inoperable ischaemic heart disease

    Active systemic infection

    Severe, irreversible hepatic disease

    Severe peripheral vascular disease

Severe obesity

Lower urinary tract dysfunction not amenable to surgical repair

Substance abuse

Significant psychiatric disturbance

*Malignancy that has been treated with no evidence of recurrence is not an exclusion criteria provided the pre-defined remission period has elapsed.

Figure 7.9 Exclusion criteria for consideration for a kidney transplant

Laboratory assessment of a potential kidney transplant recipient

Electrolytes, liver function tests, glucose, C-reactive protein

Acid-base status

Full blood count

Clotting profile

Cytomegalovirus (CMV)

Hepatitis B and C

Varicella-Zoster virus (VZV)

Epstein-Barr virus (EBV)

HIV 1 & 2

Toxoplasma

Syphilis

Blood group: ABO compatibility*

Tissue typing: human leucocyte antigen (HLA)

Panel reactive antibodies (PRA): an index of recipient reactivity to specific HLA antigens on a panel of various sample cells with known HLA type

*See text: currently transplantation across ABO barriers occurs in selected cases

Figure 7.10 Laboratory assessment of a potential kidney transplant recipient

ABO blood group incompatibility and HLA crossmatch reactivity between donor organs and recipients results in an accelerated or 'hyperacute' rejection of the non-self organ (allograft) and traditionally have been barriers to transplantation. Recent developments have led to desensitisation protocols to remove the pre-formed antibodies from the plasma of potential recipients and have permitted transplantation across ABO and HLA barriers. This has permitted previously unsuitable potential live donors to donate. Two desensitisation protocols have been employed: plasma exchange and intravenous immunoglobulin, both in conjunction with maintenance immunosuppression. The immunomodulatory effects of intravenous immunoglobulin are poorly understood. Following transplantation, clinicians and the tissue typing laboratory must remain vigilant for the persistence or reappearance of antibodies that may mediate rejection of the allograft.

The operation

The donor kidney is usually placed extraperitoneally in the right or left iliac fossa. Anastomoses are constructed joining the transplant renal artery and vein to the recipient's respective iliac vessels. The ureter is joined to the bladder. The native kidneys are left *in situ* in the majority of cases. Living donor kidneys can be retrieved either through open surgery or with the aid of laparoscopic techniques.

Postoperative period

During the initial postoperative phase of 1 to 2 weeks, careful monitoring of serum creatinine and urine output is required to assess the function of the transplanted kidney (graft). Most grafts produce measurable amounts of urine within a matter of hours and this is a clear sign of a functioning graft. However, in a certain proportion, perhaps 5 to 10% of cases, there is apparent primary non-function. Continuing dialysis support is necessary in this subgroup. In some patients the condition resolves without treatment, but in others a percutaneous kidney biopsy may be necessary to establish whether the graft is still viable and what form of therapy should be initiated. In otherwise uncomplicated cases, the serum creatinine concentration falls rapidly postoperatively and consequently changes in the rate of fall of creatinine are monitored to detect early acute rejection episodes. The differential diagnosis of graft dysfunction depends on the time since the transplant. In the very early postoperative phase this includes delayed graft function, acute vascular and cellular rejection, drug toxicity and acute tubular damage. Relative hypotension and dehydration may also contribute. Renal artery and venous thrombosis are rare complications and ureteric obstruction can be readily diagnosed using ultrasonography. Histological examination of a transplant biopsy may be necessary to aid diagnosis and adjust treatment. During acute rejection there is an interstitial cellular infiltrate, tubulitis, tubular necrosis, and a moderate or severe intimal arteritis. Unfortunately, even this approach is not completely reliable and response to treatment should be carefully monitored. Complications of kidney transplantation are summarised in Figure 7.11.

Complications following kidney transplantation

	Immediate post-transplant period	Early post-transplant period until 3 months	3-12 months	After 1 year	Comments
Surgical complications	Renal venous thrombosis. Arterial thrombosis.	Pelvic lymphocele adjacent to the transplanted kidney, ureteric obstruction, renal artery stenosis.		Ureteric obstruction, renal artery stenosis.	Increased incidence of lymphocele reported with sirolimus
Kidney	Acute tubular necrosis with delayed graft function.				Dialysis treatment may need to be continued. Transplant usually recovers following adjustment of CNI doses.
a) immunological	Hyperacute rejection: occurs as a consequence of pre-formed antibodies in recipient serum to donor blood group or HLA antigens resulting in graft failure. Plasma exchange may be initiated but transplant nephrectomy likely.	Acute rejection in 20-60% of patients. Associated with rise in serum creatinine concentration. Confirmed on biopsy. Pathological description includes vascular and cellular infiltration by immune reactive cells. Requires urgent treatment with high dose corticosteroids.	a) Chronic allograft nephropathy. Heralded by rising serum creatinine, proteinuria and hypertension. Common cause of graft failure in the long term. Complex pathogenesis with a combination of donor-specific and recipient influences. b) Subclinical rejection not suspected from serum creatinine concentration. This is a pathological diagnosis from transplant biopsy and is treated with high dose corticosteroids.		Transplant centres may perform biopsy protocols at 3, 6 and 12 months to guide therapy. Reduction in immuno-suppression during maintenance phase of stable transplants.
b) recurrent disease	Glomerular disease such as FSGS and MCGN may occur early and lead to graft failure.		Risk of anti-GBM disease in patients with Alport's syndrome. Familial haemolytic-uraemic syndrome (HUS)		Low risk of recurrent disease causing graft failure in diabetes and IgA nephropathy.

Figure 7.11 Complications following kidney transplantation

	Immediate post-transplant	Early post-transplant period until 3 months	3-12 months	After 1 year	Comments
Infection	Chest infection Urinary tract infection Septicaemia	Opportunistic infections: PCP, CMV infection and reactivation. High risk cases include donor positive and recipient negative for prior exposure to CMV (D+/R-) Prophylactic antiviral drugs recommended in high risk patients. Varicella-Zoster virus. Polyoma virus (BK virus nephropathy), candidiasis.	CMV viraemia in high risk cases following discontinuation of prophylactic anti-viral medication.		Increased risk of infection in all patients receiving immuno-suppression. Patients advised to receive influenza vaccine annually and vaccination against pneumococcus.
Drug related toxicity (see Figure 7.12)					
Lympho-proliferative		PTLD. Typically associated with EBV expression in patients exposed to highly immuno-suppressive protocols.	PTLD Includes non-EBV-related lymphoma		
Malignancy	Increased risk of non-melanotic skin malignancy and solid organ malignancy in all patients.				
Cardiovascular	Increased risk of cardiovascular disease following transplantation. Death with a functioning graft is a common cause of 'graft failure'. The majority of transplant patients require treatment for hypertension and dyslipidaemias.				

CMV, cytomegalovirus; CNI, calcineurin inhibitor; D+/R-, donor positive, recipient negative; EBV, Epstein-Barr virus; FSGS, focal segmental glomerulosclerosis; GMB, glomerular basement membrane; MCGN, mesangiocapillary glomerulonephritis; PCP, pneumocystis carineii pneumonia; PTLD, posttransplant lymphoproliferative diseases

Figure 7.11 cont. Complications following kidney transplantation

Simultaneous pancreas-kidney transplantation

Patients with type 1 diabetes and Stage 5 CKD with limited secondary complications of diabetes may be considered for simultaneous pancreas and kidney (SPK) transplantation. Patients tend to be younger than kidney only recipients and are usually aged between 20-40 years. There are 2500 patients with type 1 diabetes on the waiting list for SPK transplantation in the US. Over 90% of pancreas transplants registered until 1996 were performed in the US, but expertise is growing in other countries. Graft and patient survival rates have recently been calculated for over 3500 recipients of a SPK transplant in the US from 1994-1997 based on data reported to the United Network for Organ Sharing (UNOS) renal registry database. The 1-year graft survival was 90% and patient survival around 93%. At five years, the graft survival was in excess of 70% and patient survival 85%. These results compare favourably to cadaveric kidney-only transplantation in diabetes. The surgical technique involves whole organ pancreas transplant with the duodenal segment draining into the urinary bladder. The kidney is attached as usual to the iliac vessels and the donor ureter is inserted into the bladder separately. Alternatively the pancreas can be drained enterically. This distinction is important since there are metabolic consequences. Postoperatively, blood glucose concentrations are monitored closely and intravenous insulin is given as necessary. Exocrine pancreatic secretion can be measured in the urine. The major fear is rejection and a number of parameters are monitored including plasma glucose, amylase and lipase, and 12 or 24 hour urinary amylase. Due to high fluid, bicarbonate and electrolyte losses into the urine there is an increased need for supplementation in SPK recipients although this is usually self-limiting. A high plasma amylase is common postoperatively and may or may not signify allograft rejection. Diagnosis of pancreatic rejection in the absence of a simultaneous kidney transplant is very difficult. Signs of rejection include fever, pain, haematuria, reduction of urinary amylase and unexplained hyperglycaemia. Organ scanning and biopsy is also used. However, the function of the pancreas mirrors that of the kidney in SPK and therefore immunosuppression can be tailored to the requirements of the kidney. For patients with bladder drainage, enteric conversion may be required for refractory problems such as dehydration, metabolic acidosis, chronic urethritis due to trypsinogen activation, UTIs and recurrent reflux pancreatitis.

Immunosuppression

The rationale for the introduction of new compounds into transplantation is to increase efficacy while reducing toxicity. Currently used drugs have potentially numerous and serious side effects. For example, treatment with corticosteroids in high or prolonged doses is associated with a number of non-immune side effects such as development of diabetes mellitus, osteoporosis, skin thinning and obesity. Bone marrow suppression is the major dose limiting side effect of treatment with AZT, a drug that inhibits purine metabolism and therefore cellular proliferation. Some side effects (infections and malignancy) reflect lack of adequate immune function and are inherent in suppressing the host immune response. These side effects include pneumocystis pneumonia, cytomegalovirus infections and certain malignancies, such as skin cancer and lymphoma. Recent data has shown that the prevalence of non-melanotic skin cancer in transplant recipients at 10 years is almost 30% in the UK and 86% in Queensland, Australia (Figure 7.12).

Non-infectious complications of immunosuppressant drugs

Corticosteroids
> Diabetes, osteopenia and osteoporosis, psychosis
> Fat redistribution
> Hypertension
> Dyslipidaemia
> Cataracts

Calcineurin inhibitors (CNI)
i) Ciclosporin
> Nephrotoxicity
> Hypertension
> Neurotoxicity
> Haemolytic uraemic syndrome
> Tubular electrolyte abnormalities
> Hirsutism
> Gingival hyperplasia
> Bone pains
> Dyslipidaemia

ii) Tacrolimus
> As for ciclosporin except no hirsutism or gingival hyperplasia
> Early increased incidence of post-transplant diabetes mellitus
> Cardiomyopathy reported, particularly in children

Mycophenolate mofetil
> Abdominal pain and diarrhoea
> Myelosuppression

Sirolimus
> Lymphocele
> Thrombocytopenia
> Hyperlipidaemia

Azathioprine
> Myelosuppression*
> Severe interaction if used with allopurinol (treatment for gout)

Biological agents
i) Anti-CD25 monoclonal antibodies
> Basiliximab and daclizumab very well tolerated
> Rarely, hypersensitivity reaction

ii) Polyclonal antithymocyte globulin (ATG), antilymphocyte globulin (ALG) and monoclonal OKT3
> Increased risk of posttransplant lymphoproliferative diseases (PTLD) and infection
> Cytokine release syndromes

* The enzyme thiopurine methyltransferase (TPMT) metabolises azathioprine; the risk of myelosuppression is increased in patients with low activity of the enzyme

Figure 7.12 Non-infectious complications of immunosuppressant drugs

Following the introduction of ciclosporin there has been a dramatic increase in 1-year graft survival, although a number of important side effects have been observed. Nephrotoxicity remains a major clinical problem and may be confirmed on biopsy. Tacrolimus has a similar mechanism of action to ciclosporin on the T cell response to antigen via inhibition of the phosphatase, calcineurin. Nephrotoxicity, hypertension and post-transplant diabetes mellitus are reported with use of this very effective immunosuppressive drug. Ciclosporin and tacrolimus are classified as calcineurin inhibitors (CNI).

Newer drugs and protocols to minimise side effect profiles of corticosteroids and CNIs have recently been introduced into clinical transplantation. For example, sirolimus, a macrolide antibiotic, is an efficacious drug associated with low levels of acute rejection. In contrast to CNI, sirolimus does not cause nephrotoxicity, gingival hyperplasia or tremor. However, sirolimus is associated with a higher incidence of thrombocytopenia and hyperlipidaemia. In addition, poor wound healing and particularly damage to the lymphatic system at the time of surgery may lead to the development of fluid-filled collections called lymphoceles. These occur more frequently with sirolimus use. Lymphoceles occasionally lead to obstruction of the transplanted kidney. Needle aspiration under radiological guidance is successful in most cases, although surgery and internalisation of the lymphocele into the peritoneal cavity may be necessary in refractory cases. MMF blocks purine metabolism, but is more potent and possibly more specific for lymphocytes than AZT. Many centres now favour MMF over AZT to prevent acute rejection in cases where there is evidence of nephrotoxicity from CNI (guidelines for use have been published by NICE in 2004 and 2006). Studies have also shown that sirolimus in combination with MMF is safe and associated with low rates of acute transplant rejection at 12 months. MMF is non-nephrotoxic.

Polyclonal antilymphocyte globulin (ALG), antithymocyte globulin (ATG) and monoclonal (OKT3) anti-T-cell antibodies, so-called 'biological agents', are available for clinical use to prevent graft rejection. They may also be used for treating an episode of acute rejection that has not responded to high dose corticosteroids and adjustment of immunosuppressive drugs. There is a high risk of opportunistic infections and lymphoproliferative diseases with these particular antibody therapies. Selective targeting of activated T cells is now feasible with the introduction of anti-CD25 antibodies (dacluzimab and basiliximab). Anti-CD25 antibodies are now used routinely in the induction and early post-operative period.

THERAPEUTIC DRUG MONITORING
Ciclosporin is insoluble and is presented for clinical use as an oral microemulsion. It has a narrow therapeutic window and it is important to monitor the blood concentration frequently. The most widely accepted practice is to monitor the

'trough' blood concentration (C0) just prior to the next dose. Accepted trough concentrations range from 100-200 μg/L with higher concentrations for the induction phase of treatment. The trough concentration within the blood may not give a truly accurate guide to total drug exposure, since there is a wide variation in bioavailability over the first 2-4 hours following oral dosing. This is important since most of the pharmacodynamic effects of ciclosporin occur within two hours. Studies from Canada suggest that trough concentrations do not reflect clinical outcomes in terms of acute rejection rates although high trough concentrations are associated with increased nephrotoxicity. A two hour drug (C2) concentration correlates well with formal area under the curve (AUC) measurements and is predictive of nephrotoxicity and acute rejection episodes. However, due to the logistic problems involved in accurately collecting a blood sample at C2 the practice has not become widely adopted in the UK. In kidney transplant patients, the trough level of tacrolimus is well correlated with acute rejection episodes and nephrotoxicity. Trough concentrations also guide sirolimus therapy. It is mandatory to perform therapeutic drug monitoring when using ciclosporin, tacrolimus and sirolimus. Weekly measurements are required in the first months following a transplant to ensure efficacy and to avoid toxicity. During the maintenance phase of a transplant the frequency of monitoring is reduced, and the interval between checks may be 3 months in long-term, stable patients. When a dose adjustment is made, it takes several days for the new steady state to be reached and a further check in one week is made. Important pharmacokinetic interactions can occur with these drugs. For example, patients are informed that concurrent ingestion of grapefruit juice with oral ciclosporin, tacrolimus and sirolimus significantly increases their bioavailability. Commonly used drugs such as the macrolide antibiotics (erythromycin and clarithromycin) and antifungal agents such as fluconazole, inhibit the metabolism of CNIs and sirolimus leading to high trough blood concentrations and potential toxicity. This combination of drugs should be avoided where possible.

MMF is the prodrug of mycophenolic acid (MPA), a selective, non-competitive inhibitor of inosine 5-monophosphate dehydrogenase, the rate-limiting step for guanosine triphosphate synthesis. Inhibition of *de novo* purine synthesis and guanosine nucleotide depletion reduces T and B lymphocyte proliferation. Although MPA can be measured in blood samples, recent data from a randomised trial of Fixed Dose therapy compared to Concentration Controlled (FDCC-trial) suggest that therapeutic drug monitoring is not necessary to reach target MPA exposure. Currently, routine measurement of MPA concentration is not recommended in kidney transplantation.

Further reading

British National Formulary 56. Section 8.2 September 2008. BMJ Publishing Group Ltd and RPS publishing.

Churchill DN, Taylor DW, Keshaviah PR for CANUSA study group. Adequacy of dialysis and nutrition in continuous peritoneal dialysis: Association with clinical outcomes. J Am Soc Nephrol 1996; **7**: 198–207.

Eknoyan G, Beck GJ, Cheung AK, Daugirdas JT, Greene T, Kusek JW *et al.* for the Hemodialysis (HEMO) Study Group. Effect of dialysis dose and membrane flux in maintenance hemodialysis. N Engl J Med 2002; **347**: 2010-9.

Kemp HJ, Parnham A, Tomson CR. Urea kinetic modelling: a measure of dialysis adequacy. Ann Clin Biochem 2001; **38**: 20-7.

National Kidney Foundation. KDOQI Clinical Practice Guidelines and Clinical Practice Recommendations for 2006 Updates: Hemodialysis Adequacy, Peritoneal Dialysis Adequacy and Vascular Access. Am J Kidney Dis 2006; **48**: S1-S322.

Pasten S, Bailey J. Dialysis therapy. N Engl J Med 1998; **338**: 1428-37.

Chapter 8

Renal service delivery: quality standards and assessment

Organisation of renal services

Background

Traditionally, services for people with ESRD have centred around dialysis facilities in a limited number of tertiary referral centres where renal consultants, in-patient and investigative facilities are based. Some of these centres also offer kidney transplantation with life-long follow-up for patients to maximise the quality of their care. This centralisation allowed expertise to develop in relatively few centres. In the 1970s and 1980s, programmes of home HD and PD were established and dialysis facilities were made available in district general hospitals in provincial cities. In the 1990s, 'hub and spoke' models developed with main renal units supported by satellite units closer to patients' homes. In the Western world, the provision of support for ESRD has expanded enormously in the last 20 years; for example, in the UK the total number of patients receiving RRT increased from 396 per million people in 1992 to 547 per million people in 2001. Around half of these patients had a functioning transplant, with the remainder being treated by dialysis. The costs of RRT are significant consuming 1-2% of the entire NHS budget, with the average annual cost of HD in a satellite unit in 2006 being £21,000 per patient. Increased provision is being matched by a similar increase in need, partly as a consequence of the ageing population and the increased prevalence of diabetes mellitus. RRT is underpinned by standards of care defined by expert bodies such as the Renal Association in the UK and NKF-KDOQI in the US, as described below.

While only 0.2% of the population has ESRD, it is increasingly recognised that CKD affects a much larger proportion of the population and, as discussed in earlier chapters, although such patients may not necessarily progress to ESRD, they are at greatly increased risk of death from cardiovascular disease. In recent years, there has been a shift in emphasis in clinical nephrology towards identification and management of the earlier stages of CKD. This has been prompted by the recognition that late referral to nephrology services in advanced CKD is associated with poor outcome. Government bodies have recognised the increasing significance of the burden of CKD, which has resulted in the development of expert clinical guidelines to assist CKD management. In this chapter, we will briefly review some of these standards and guidelines, with particular reference to those emanating from the UK and their interaction with laboratory medicine. More detailed information may be found on websites supported by the professional bodies cited.

National Service Framework (NSF) for Renal Services

While the UK government has invested considerably in expanding capacity for treating people with ESRD, there is recognition that there remains an unmet need, particularly for HD among older people. It is also clear that treatment rates for ESRD are lower in the UK than in other comparable countries and that there is a variation in treatment rates in different parts of the UK, not fully explained by demographic differences. Against this background, the Department of Health in England developed the NSF for Renal Services which aims to build on current models of service provision and develop renal networks providing integrated care closer to patients' homes and equity of access. The NSF was published in two stages, with Part One (published 2004) focusing on dialysis and transplantation and Part Two (published 2005) on CKD, ARF and end of life care.

NATIONAL SERVICE FRAMEWORK FOR RENAL SERVICES: PART ONE

In Part One of the NSF, five standards of care were set with 30 underpinning markers of good practice that could be subjected to audit. While lacking in explicit recommendations for laboratory practice, the NSF clearly recognises the importance of diagnostic services, including pathology, as part of an integrated renal service. For example, standard five, concerning kidney transplant services, has an underpinning marker of good practice that states: 'Appropriate immunosuppression and antirejection treatment in accordance with … NICE guidance and effective monitoring and treatment to minimise the risks of adverse effects of immuno-suppressive treatment'. Standard two, relating to preparation for, and choice of dialysis treatment, identifies management of anaemia to maintain an adequate haemoglobin concentration. Throughout the NSF there is an emphasis on integration with other NSFs (e.g. those for diabetes, older people and coronary heart disease) and NICE guidance (e.g. those for home versus hospital HD, the detection and management of diabetic renal disease and hypertension, and the subsequently published NICE guidance on immunosuppressive therapy and anaemia management). Explicitly, all renal and transplant units were urged to participate in national comparative audit and benchmarking by submitting data to the UK Renal Registry (see below).

NATIONAL SERVICE FRAMEWORK FOR RENAL SERVICES: PART TWO

Part Two of the Renal NSF identifies four quality requirements covering CKD, ARF and end of life care. Quality requirements one and two are concerned with prevention and early detection of CKD and minimising the progression and consequences of CKD. To achieve these aims, there is a requirement that people at increased risk of CKD (e.g. those with diabetes, hypertension or cardiovascular disease) should have their kidney function assessed. Explicitly, it is recommended that the 'at risk' population should have their urine screened for proteinuria by measuring a protein:creatinine ratio on a random sample and that the blood test of kidney function should be an estimated GFR, calculated and reported automatically by all clinical biochemistry laboratories. The need for integrated care across the primary and secondary care interface is recognised, with referral to specialist services at an appropriate stage to optimise outcomes. In particular, there is an emphasis on optimal management of blood pressure, particularly using ACE inhibitors and ARBs, diabetic control, cardiovascular disease, renal bone disease, urinary tract obstruction and infection. Clearly this is a complex area of medicine and the NSF, with its emphasis on policy direction, was never likely to provide detailed guidance. Guidelines for the identification, management and referral of adults with CKD have been developed by a multidisciplinary group to underpin the recommendations of the NSF and are discussed later in this chapter (p208).

The UK Renal Association: standards, guidelines and audit

The Renal Association (www.renal.org), founded in 1950, is the UK professional body for nephrologists and renal scientists. It is active in the planning and development of renal services and nephrology in Britain and in the promotion and dissemination of research and education relating to the specialty. The Clinical Practice Guidelines Committee of the Renal Association prepares standards ('guidelines') for the UK renal community. These in turn define the data collected by the UK Renal Registry, which is itself a committee of the UK Renal Association.

The Renal Association clinical practice guidelines provide a template for the management of patients with kidney disease in the UK. The 1st edition of the standards document was produced in 1995. The current (4th) edition was published on-line in modules between 2007 and 2008. Hitherto, the standards document had primarily concerned itself with ESRD patients. The current version was written as five separate modules addressing CKD, complications, dialysis, transplantation and ARF. Reflecting terminology used by other groups, the term 'standards' has been dropped in favour of 'clinical practice guidelines'.

In addition to standards relating to dialysis and transplantation facilities and access, there are many standards directly relevant to laboratory practice. Some of these have been discussed in earlier chapters of this book, for example those relating to PTH and management of anaemia (Chapter 6). Additionally, there are standards relating to microbiological surveillance, dialysis adequacy, management of cardiovascular risk and nutrition. It is not our intention to reproduce the standards document here but for illustration, laboratory indices of haemodialysis adequacy are shown in Figure 8.1.

Laboratory indices of haemodialysis adequacy

Blood sampling for biochemical and haematological measurements should be performed before a mid-week haemodialysis session using a dry needle or syringe.

Monitoring of predialysis biochemical and haematological parameters should be performed monthly in hospital haemodialysis patients and at least three-monthly in home haemodialysis patients.

- Pre-dialysis serum bicarbonate concentrations, measured with minimum delay after venepuncture, should be between 20 and 26 mmol/L.

- Pre-dialysis serum potassium concentration should be between 3.5 and 6.5 mmol/L.

- Pre-dialysis serum phosphate concentration should be between 1.1 and 1.8 mmol/L.

- Pre-dialysis serum calcium concentration, adjusted for serum albumin, should be within the normal range, preferably below 2.5 mmol/L.

- Pre-dialysis serum corrected calcium x phosphate product should be less than 4.8 $mmol^2/L^2$.

- Serum PTH concentration should be more than twice and less than four times the upper limit of normal for the intact PTH assay used.

- Serum aluminium concentration should be measured every three months in all patients receiving oral aluminium hydroxide.

- Pre-dialysis haemoglobin concentration should be greater than 10 g/dL.

Figure 8.1. Laboratory indices of haemodialysis adequacy (other than dialysis dose). Reproduced with permission from the UK Renal Association Clinical Practice Guidelines 4th edition, 2007).

It would behove all staff working in laboratories supporting renal units to gain an understanding of the framework against which renal units monitor their patients' condition. Figure 8.2 details the kind of laboratory support that is required by a typical renal unit.

Laboratory support for a renal replacement therapy programme

Clinical situation	Laboratory tests
Acute complications	
Dialysis disequilibrium	Serum electrolytes
Pyrexia	Serum CRP
Bleeding	Clotting factors
Chronic complications	
Anaemia	Blood haemoglobin, serum ferritin, serum folate
Septicaemia/peritonitis	Serum CRP, blood culture and sensitivity
Malnutrition	Serum albumin
Cardiovascular disease	Serum lipid profile
Osteodystrophy	Serum calcium, phosphate, alkaline phosphatase, PTH, aluminium
Immunity monitoring	HBsAG, HCV antibody, HIV antibody
Adequacy of dialysis	
Urea kinetic modelling (URR)	Pre- and post-dialysis urea
Weekly creatinine clearances	Pre- and post-dialysis creatinine
Peritoneal equilibration test (PET)	Serum/plasma and dialysate creatinine and glucose
Transplant Monitoring	
Immunosuppression	Trough (or 2 h) whole blood ciclosporin, tacrolimus and sirolimus
Graft function	Serum creatinine, serum and urine electrolytes

Figure 8.2. Laboratory support for a renal replacement therapy programme.

Other organisations internationally have also developed clinical practice guidelines for kidney disease. In the USA, the National Kidney Foundation K/DOQI has produced a series of guidelines covering aspects of ESRD care and CKD detection and management (www.kidney.org/professionals/KDOQI/guidelines.cfm). This work was begun in 1997 and regular updates of the guidelines are hosted on the organisation's website. In Australasia, Kidney Health Australia and the Australian and New Zealand Society of Nephrology have published the CARI (Caring for Australasians with Renal Impairment) Guidelines (www.kidney.org.au). European Best Practice Guidelines (www.era-edta.org/ebpg.htm) and Canadian Society of Nephrology guidelines (www.csnscn.ca/english/home/default.asp?s=1) are also available.

The UK Renal Registry

The UK Renal Registry was established by the Renal Association with support from the Department of Health, the British Association of Paediatric Nephrologists and the British Transplant Society, to act as a resource in the development of patient care in renal disease. The Renal Association standards ('guidelines') document includes audit measures that are monitored by the Renal Registry, thus enabling the Registry to act as a source of comparative data for benchmarking, planning, policy and research. The data include biochemical and haematological parameters that are collected quarterly by automatic downloading from all participating renal unit databases in England, Wales and Northern Ireland. (There is a separate Scottish Renal Registry, although it does provide demographic data from the whole of Scotland to the UK Renal Registry). The Registry is funded from commissioning agencies by a capitation fee on renal patients and captures data from over 90% of the UK dialysis and transplantation population. In addition to laboratory data, the Registry collects a variety of other data, including prevalence of and access to RRT, causes of ESRD, RRT modality and survival of patients on RRT.

Much of the annual report is devoted to analysis of performance at individual renal centre level against the Renal Association standards. This enables nephrologists to compare the performance of their own unit and, in some cases, identify and address deficiencies. For example, the Renal Association standard for phosphate control states: 'serum phosphate (measured before a dialysis session in a haemodialysis patient) should be between 1.1 and 1.8 mmol/L'. It is clear from Figure 8.3 that there is wide variation in the attainment of this target between dialysis units and that, generally, performance against this target is poor, with only approximately 55% of patients achieving the target. The Registry database also permits exploratory analyses that can look at trends. For example, with regard to serum phosphate, it has been possible to show that there has been a year-on-year improvement in phosphate control within both the haemodialysis and peritoneal dialysis populations (Figure 8.4). The annual report is freely available on the website of the UK Renal Registry (www.renalreg.com).

Percentage of haemodialysis patients achieving phosphate targets

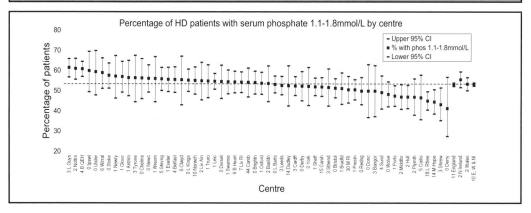

Figure 8.3 Percentage of haemodialysis patients achieving the Renal Association target for serum phosphate concentration (1.1 - 1.8 mmol/L) in 2007. Data are presented for individual renal units with the mean attainment for all patients in England and Wales shown on the right of the figure. Reproduced with permission of the UK Renal Registry.

Percentage of haemodialysis patients achieving phosphate targets

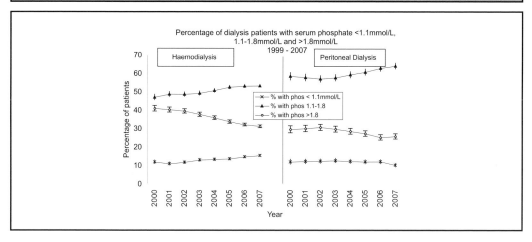

Figure 8.4 Percentage of dialysis patients in England and Wales achieving the UK Renal Association target for serum phosphate control (1.1 - 1.8 mmol/L) over the period 2000 to 2007. The left hand panel shows haemodialysis patients and the right hand panel peritoneal dialysis patients. It can be seen that achievement of the target has generally improved over this period and that control is better among peritoneal dialysis than haemodialysis patients. Reproduced with permission of the UK Renal Registry.

Chronic kidney disease guidelines

UK guidelines for the identification, management and referral of patients with CKD have been developed at the suggestion of the Joint Specialty Committee on Renal Disease of the Royal College of Physicians of London and the Renal Association, although a variety of other professional groups, including the Association for Clinical Biochemistry, were involved in their development. Similar guidelines have been developed by other national professional bodies and can be found on the websites referred to above. The UK guidelines published in 2006 were specifically developed to promote the optimal management of CKD within the NHS setting and were developed in parallel with, but independently from, part two of the NSF for Renal Services. The guidelines primarily address two questions:

1) how should people with CKD be identified in the NHS?

2) what is the optimum method of management and referral of patients with CKD?

The guidelines clearly defined who should be screened for CKD, how secondary complications should be managed and monitored and when patients should be referred for specialist nephrology care (www.renal.org/CKDguide/full/CKDprintedfullguide.pdf). While aspects of the guidelines proved controversial in the laboratory community (for example, recommendations concerning the detection of renal osteodystrophy) especially since many of the recommendations were based on expert opinion rather than randomised controlled trials, the guidelines provided a framework ensuring a consistent and rational approach to the management of CKD across the UK.

In September 2008, NICE published a clinical practice guideline relating to the early identification and management of adults with CKD in primary and secondary care (www.nice.org.uk/guidance/index.jsp?action=byID&o=12069). This guideline builds upon, and effectively supersedes, the earlier UK CKD guidelines. Several important changes have been recommended by the NICE guidance. Perhaps the most significant from the laboratory perspective is the recommendation that reagent strip devices should not be used for the detection of proteinuria. In both diabetic and non-diabetic individuals, urinary albumin:creatinine ratio should be used in preference to protein:creatinine ratio, on the basis of its greater sensitivity for low level proteinuria. This represents an important effort to reconcile differences in the approach to investigation between the diabetic and non-diabetic specialties and should simplify understanding of proteinuria among non-specialists. In non-diabetic individuals, significant proteinuria is defined as an albumin:creatinine ratio of 30 mg/mmol or greater. There is also a recommendation that stage 3 CKD in the international classification of CKD (Figure 2.2) should be subdivided into two sub-stages: 3A (GFR 45-59 mL/min/1.73 m^2) and 3B (GFR 30-44 mL/min/1.73 m^2), on the basis of their differing epidemiological and prognostic significance, and that the suffix 'p' should be used at all stages to denote the presence of proteinuria. The use of estimated GFR has been reinforced, with clear recommendations relating to which individuals should be tested (Figure 8.5) and how often, which equation should be used with which creatinine assays, in addition to guidance relating to pre-analytical influences. The guidelines offer important advice relating to the laboratory monitoring of individuals receiving ACE inhibitor/ARB treatment. The recommendation that routine measurement of calcium, phosphate, PTH and vitamin D concentrations in people with stages 1 to 3 CKD is not indicated may be welcomed by some members of the laboratory community.

As discussed above, the Renal NSF made a clear statement that estimated GFR and urinary protein:creatinine ratio should be used as tools to detect CKD in the at risk population. As an incentive to maximise the effectiveness of the NSF roll-out, a renal domain was included in the Quality and Outcomes Framework (QOF) of the General Medical Services Contract from 1st April 2006. This is a payment scheme for primary care physicians, which may represent up to 40% of practice income. Four renal criteria were initially set and primary care practices were asked to establish a register of patients with CKD (GFR < 60 mL/min/1.73 m^2). Among the patients thus identified, further points are awarded depending on how many have had a blood pressure recording, how many have a blood pressure below 140/85 mmHg and how many are being treated with renin-angiotensin blockade. Overall, 27 points were initially available for the CKD domain, of a total of approximately 600 points in the QOF. From 2009, a fifth criteria relating to proteinuria measurement was included.

The great majority of patients starting RRT have progressed from earlier stages of CKD. Most could therefore have been identified earlier, with possible improvements in outcome. Although ESRD is relatively rare, treatment with dialysis or transplantation is very expensive. Any improvement in the early identification and management of CKD is therefore highly desirable. Recent years have seen kidney disease move up the health-political agenda in the UK. With the publication of the Renal NSF and NICE guidelines in England and Wales and of the Scottish Intercollegiate Guideline Network (SIGN) guideline in Scotland, supplemented with incentivisation through the QOF, the importance of kidney disease as a major public health issue is now firmly established in the UK.

Early identification of CKD

Offer testing for CKD if there are any of the following risk factors:

- diabetes

- hypertension

- cardiovascular disease (ischaemic heart disease, chronic heart failure, peripheral vascular disease and cerebral vascular disease)

- structural renal tract disease, renal calculi or prostatic hypertrophy

- multisystem diseases with potential kidney involvement, e.g. systemic lupus erythematosus

- family history of stage 5 CKD or hereditary kidney disease

- opportunistic detection of haematuria or proteinuria.

In the absence of the above risk factors, do not use age, gender or ethnicity as risk markers to test people for CKD. In the absence of metabolic syndrome, diabetes or hypertension, do not use obesity alone as a risk marker to test people for CKD.

Monitor GFR in people prescribed drugs known to be nephrotoxic, such as calcineurin inhibitors and lithium. Check GFR at least annually in people receiving long-term systemic non-steroidal anti-inflammatory drug treatment.

Figure 8.5 Early identification of CKD. Reproduced from the NICE CKD Guideline (CG 73).

Further reading

Department of Health. The National Service Framework for Renal Services Part 1: Dialysis and Transplantation. 2004: www.dh.gov.uk/PolicyAndGuidance/HealthAndSocialCareTopics/ Renal/fs/en (accessed 26th January 2009).

Department of Health. The National Service Framework for Renal Services Part 2: Chronic Kidney Disease, Acute Renal Failure and End of life Care. 2005: www.dh.gov.uk/PolicyAndGuidance/HealthAndSocialCareTopics/ Renal/fs/en (accessed 26th January 2009).

Joint Specialty Committee on Renal Medicine of the Royal College of Physicians and the Renal Association and the Royal College of General Practitioners. Chronic Kidney Disease in Adults: UK Guidelines for Identification, Management and Referral. London: Royal College of Physicians, 2006: www.renal.org/CKDguide/full/CKDprintedfullguide.pdf (accessed 26th January 2009).

National Institute for Health and Clinical Excellence. Chronic Kidney Disease. Early identification and management of chronic kidney disease in adults in primary and secondary care (Clinical Guideline 73) 2008: www.nice.org.uk/guidance/index.jsp?action=byID&o=12069 (accessed 26th January 2009).

Renal Association. Clinical Practice Guidelines 4th Edition 2007-8: www.renal.org (accessed 26th January 2009).

Scottish Intercollegiate Guideline Network (SIGN). Diagnosis and Management of Chronic Kidney Disease (Guideline 103) 2008: www.sign.ac.uk/guidelines/fulltext/103/index.html (accessed 26th January 2009)

UK Renal Registry Reports, Bristol, UK. Reports are published annually: www.renalreg.com (accessed 26th January 2009).

List of abbreviations

$1,25(OH_2)D_3$	calcitriol
11β-HSD	11β-hydroxysteroid dehydrogenase
^{99}mTc-DMSA	^{99}mTc-dimercaptosuccinic acid
^{99}mTc-DTPA	^{99}mTc-diethylenetriaminepentaacetic acid
^{99}mTc-MAG3	^{99}mTc-mercaptoacetyltriglycerine
AII	angiotensin II
ACE	angiotensin converting enzyme
ACP	acute coronary syndrome
ADH	antidiuretic hormone
ADPKD	autosomal dominant polycystic kidney disease
AE1	anion exchanger 1
AGE	advanced glycation end products
AIN	acute interstitial nephritis
ALG	anti-lymphocyte globulin
ALP	alkaline phosphatase
ANA	antinuclear antibodies
ANCA	anti-neutrophil cytoplasmic antibody
ANP	atrial natriuretic peptide
anti GBM	antiglomerular basement membrane
APD	automated peritoneal dialysis
AQP	aquaporins
ARB	angiotensin receptor blocker
ARF	acute renal failure
ARAS	atheromatous renal artery stenosis
ARPKD	autosomal recessive polycystic kidney disease
ATN	acute tubular necrosis
AVF	arteriovenous fistula
AZT	azathioprine
BJP	Bence Jones protein
BMI	body mass index
BP	blood pressure
BSA	body surface area
CAII	carbonic anhydrase II
CAIV	carbonic anhydrase IV
CAN	chronic allograft nephropathy
CAPD	continuous ambulatory peritoneal dialysis
CFU	colony forming units
CHD	coronary heart disease
CKD	chronic kidney disease

CLC-Kb	basolateral chloride channel
CNI	calcineurin inhibitors
COL4A5	A5 chain of type IV collagen
CRP	C-reactive protein
CT	computed tomography
CO_2	carbon dioxide
CRF	chronic renal failure
CVP	central venous pressure
CyA	ciclosporin A
dRTA	distal renal tubular acidosis
DCCT	Diabetes Control and Complications Trial
DTPA	^{99}mTc-diethylenetriaminepentaacetic acid
DVT	deep vein thrombosis
EDTA	ethylenediaminetetraacetic acid
EM	electron microscopy
ENaC	apical sodium channel
EMU	early morning urine
EPO	erythropoietin
ERF	established renal failure
ESAs	erythropoiesis stimulating agents
ESRD	end-stage renal disease
ESWL	extracorporeal shock wave lithotripsy
FENa	fractional excretion of sodium
FSGS	focal segmental glomerulosclerosis
GBM	glomerular basement membrane
GFR	glomerular filtration rate
GN	glomerulonephritis
GSC	glomerular sieving coefficient
H_2CO_3	carbonic acid
HDF	haemodiafiltration
HD	haemodialysis
HF	haemofiltration
HIV	human immunodeficiency virus
HLA	human leucocyte antigen
HOT	Hypertension Optimal Treatment
HPLC	high performance liquid chromatography
ID-MS	isotope dilution mass spectrometry
Ig	immunoglobulin
IM	immunoperoxidase
IVP	intravenous pyelography
IVU	intravenous urography

JGA	juxtaglomerular apparatus
JNC-VII	Joint National Committee on Prevention, Detection, Evaluation, and Treatment of High Blood Pressure
K/DOQI	Kidney Disease Outcomes Quality Initiative
LCDD	light chain deposition disease
LM	light microscopy
MCD	minimal change disease
MCGN	mesangiocapillary glomerulonephritis
MDRD	Modification of Diet in Renal Disease
MHC	major histocompatibility complex
MMF	mycophenolate mofetil
6-MP	6-mercaptopurine
MPA	mycophenolic acid
MRA	magnetic resonance angiography
MRI	magnetic resonance imaging
MR	mineralocorticoid receptor
NBC-1	Na^+-HCO_3^- cotransporter
Na^+-K^+-ATPase	sodium-potassium adenosine triphosphatase
NAG	N-acetyl-β-D-glucosaminidase
NBC-1	Na^+-HCO_3^- cotransporter
NCCT	Na^+-Cl^- cotransporter
NCXl	sodium calcium exchanger
NHANES III	Third National Health and Nutrition Examination Survey
NHS	National Health Service
NHE-3	Na^+-H^+ exchanger
NICE	National Institute for Health and Clinical Excellence
NKCC2	Na^+-K^+-2Cl^- cotransporter
NKF-K/DOQI	National Kidney Foundation – Kidney Disease Outcomes Quality Initiative
NSAIDs	non-steroidal anti-inflammatory drugs
NSF	National Service Framework
PD	peritoneal dialysis
PET	peritoneal equilibration test
pRTA	proximal renal tubular acidosis
PKC-β1	protein kinase C-β1
pmp	per million population
PTH	parathyroid hormone
pIgA	polymeric IgA
QOF	Quality and Outcomes Framework
RAAS	renin-angiotensin-aldosterone system
rhEPO	recombinant human erythropoietin

RBP	retinol binding protein
RIFLE	Risk, Injury, Failure, Loss, End-stage kidney disease
RPGN	rapidly progressive glomerulonephritis
RRF	residual renal function
RRT	renal replacement therapy
RTA	renal tubular acidosis
RVT	renal vein thrombosis
SAP	serum amyloid protein
SGA	subjective global assessment
SIGN	Scottish Intercollegiate Guideline Network
SLE	systemic lupus erythematosus
SPK	simultaneous pancreas and kidney
TGF-β	transforming growth factor beta
THG	Tamm Horsfall glycoprotein
TNF-α	tissue necrosis factor-α
Tm	tubular maximal uptake
TMB	tetramethyl benzidine
UF	ultrafiltration
UK	United Kingdom
UKNEQAS	United Kingdom National External Quality Assessment Scheme
UKPDS	United Kingdom Prospective Diabetes Study
UKM	urea kinetic modelling
UKT	UK transplant
UNOS	United Network for Organ Sharing
URR	urea reduction ratio
US	United States
USRDS	United States Renal Data System
UTI	urinary tract infection

ACB Venture Publications
Calculations in Laboratory Medicine
by Allan Deacon
Edited by Roy Sherwood & James Hooper

Due 2009 £35

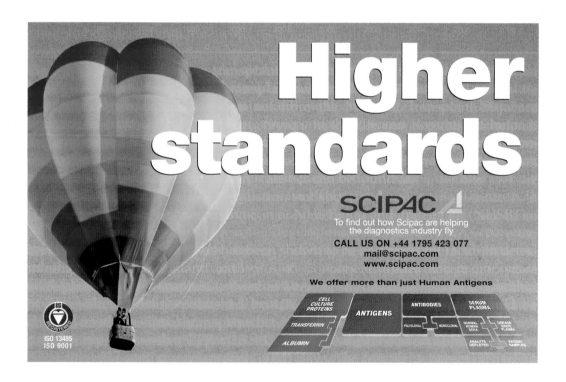

Higher standards

SCIPAC

To find out how Scipac are helping the diagnostics industry fly

CALL US ON +44 1795 423 077
mail@scipac.com
www.scipac.com

We offer more than just Human Antigens

ISO 13485
ISO 9001

CELL CULTURE PROTEINS

TRANSFERRIN

ALBUMIN

ANTIGENS

ANTIBODIES

POLYCLONAL   MONOCLONAL

SERUM PLASMA

NORMAL HUMAN SERA

ANALYTE DEPLETED

DISEASE STATE PLASMA

PATIENT SAMPLES